Data Interpretation Made Easy

For medical students and junior doctors

NEEL SHARMA

Foreword by

TIAGO VILLANUEVA

General Practitioner
Former BMJ *Clegg Scholar*
Past Editor of the Student BMJ

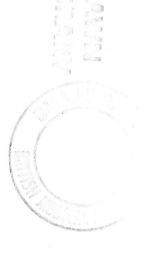

Radcliffe Publishing
London • New York

Radcliffe Publishing Ltd
33–41 Dallington Street
London
EC1V 0BB
United Kingdom

www.radcliffehealth.com

British Library Cataloguing in Publication Data

A catalogue record for this book is available from the British Library.

ISBN-13: 978 184619 329 3

The paper used for the text pages of this book
is FSC® certified. FSC (The Forest Stewardship
Council®) is an international network to promote
responsible management of the world's forests.

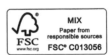

Typeset by Darkriver Design, Auckland, New Zealand
Printed and bound by TJI Digital, Padstow, Cornwall, UK

Contents

Foreword

No matter how proficient you are at patient history-taking or physical examination, practicing modern medicine to high standards also entails analysing and integrating a sobering amount of laboratory and radiological types of data. The information obtained through these tests is often pivotal, as it allows doctors to clinch the right diagnosis and to guide subsequent treatment decisions. Clinical reasoning has become more complex than ever, and medical training and continuous medical education must keep up with these increasing demands.

Dr Neel Sharma's latest venture on data interpretation has dozens of credible clinical scenarios covering many key areas of clinical medicine. And you will certainly feel challenged, as he leaves it up to you to diagnose and devise the treatment plan.

Dr Tiago Villanueva
General Practitioner
Former *BMJ* Clegg Scholar
Past Editor of the *Student BMJ*
May 2013

Preface

As doctors, the ability to interpret and synthesise medical data is essential – a skill that takes time to develop and is often not so straightforward to master, even for experienced doctors.

This book focuses purely on developing this skill through the inclusion of blood results, X-rays and ECGs allied to a variety of medical presentations. And all cases described are complemented with evidence-based practice, ensuring its worth for students and junior doctors.

One thing I would like to point out is that I have deliberately made the case histories short to emphasise the focus of this book, as the practice of medicine is never textbook based, something I appreciated during my early years as a doctor.

And, of course, I am more than happy to answer any queries based on the material provided, so please feel free to contact me at n.sharma@qmul.ac.uk or through direct contact with Radcliffe Publishing.

I sincerely hope you find this book useful and wish you all the success in your future careers.

Dr Neel Sharma
Honorary Tutor
Institute of Medical and Health Sciences Education
Li Ka Shing Faculty of Medicine
The University of Hong Kong
and
Clinical Lecturer
Centre for Medical Education
Barts and the London School of Medicine and Dentistry
May 2013

About the author

Neel graduated from Manchester University with bachelor degrees in Pharmacology and Medicine. He also holds an MSc in Gastroenterology from Barts and the London School of Medicine and Dentistry.

Neel undertook his foundation and core medical training in London and maintains a strong interest in medical education. He was appointed Clinical Lecturer at the Centre for Medical Education at Barts in 2011, and is currently a Tutor at the Institute of Medical and Health Sciences Education, Li Ka Shing Faculty of Medicine, the University of Hong Kong. He is also a member of the Curriculum Development Team for the newly established Lee Kong Chian School of Medicine in Singapore.

Contributor

Cardiology cases: Dr Faezeh Godazgar, Foundation Doctor, North West Thames

I would like to dedicate this book to my parents,
Ravi and Anita, and my sister, Ravnita.
Without their continued support and encouragement
none of this would have truly been possible.

1

Cardiology

Case 1

You are bleeped to see a 54-year-old man on the medical ward. A nurse has performed the following ECG and asks you to review it:

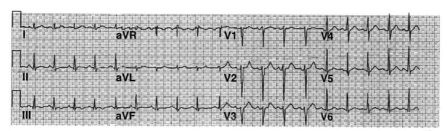

Q. What management plan would you instigate in view of the ECG?

Case 2

You are asked to review the following ECG by a nurse. The ECG is shown below:

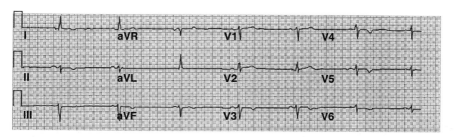

Q. What management plan would you instigate in view of the ECG?

Case 3

You are asked to review the following ECG:

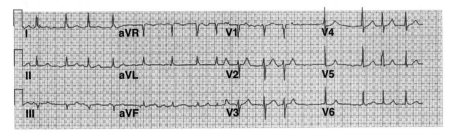

Q. What management plan would you instigate in view of the above ECG?

Case 4

A 45-year-old man presents to Accident and Emergency (A and E) with dizzy spells. Past medical history reveals hypertension, for which he takes atenolol. Routine observations demonstrate a heart rate of 55 beats per minute, blood pressure of 80/55 mmHg and oxygen saturations of 98% on room air. An ECG is performed, which is shown below:

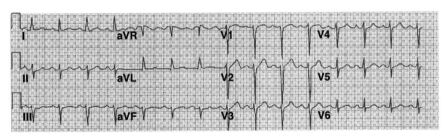

Q. What management plan would you instigate in view of the ECG?

Case 5

You are asked to review a patient's ECG whilst on call. The patient was admitted with shortness of breath and was treated for a chest infection. He has a past medical history of atrial fibrillation, for which he takes digoxin. The ECG is shown below:

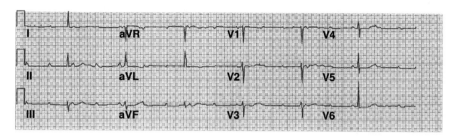

Q. What management plan would you instigate in view of the ECG?

Case 6

A 45-year-old man is admitted with central crushing chest pain. He has a past medical history of ischaemic heart disease and hypertension. An ECG is performed, which is shown below:

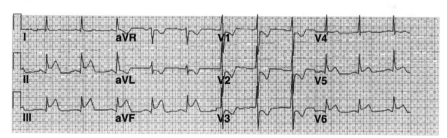

Q. What management plan would you instigate in view of the ECG?

Case 7

A 45-year-old woman presents to A and E with chest pain and visual disturbance. She has a past medical history of atrial fibrillation, for which she takes digoxin. An ECG is performed, which is shown below:

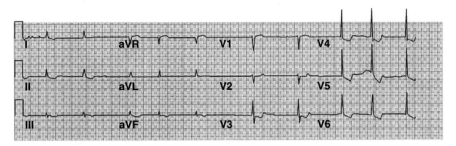

Q. What management plan would you instigate?

Case 8

A 65-year-old man is admitted with central chest pain. Three weeks previously he was treated for a myocardial infarction. An ECG is performed, which is shown below:

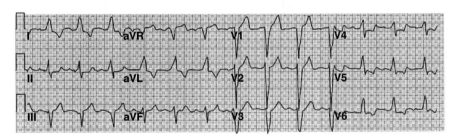

Q. What does the ECG show?

Case 9

A 43-year-old woman is admitted to A and E with dizzy spells. She has a past medical history of Type II diabetes, for which she takes metformin. Routine observations demonstrate a blood pressure of 176/86 mmHg and pulse rate of 98 beats per minute. An ECG is performed, which is shown below:

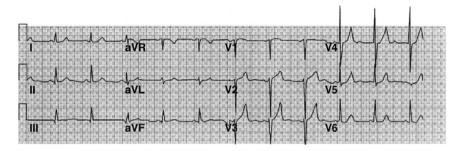

Q. What management plan would you instigate?

Case 10

You are an FY1 on call when you are paged to see a patient. On arrival you note the patient is unresponsive and has no pulse. The nurse commences chest compressions while you attach a defibrillator. The following rhythm strip is noted:

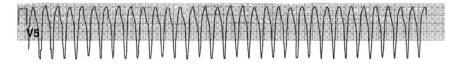

Q. What management plan would you instigate?

Case 11

You are an FY2 on call when you are asked to review a patient complaining of chest pain. An ECG is performed, which is shown below:

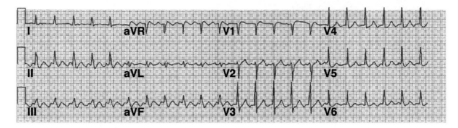

Q. What management plan would you instigate?

Case 12

A 65-year-old man presents to A and E with palpitations. An ECG is performed, which is shown below:

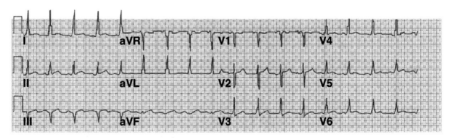

Q. What management plan would you instigate?

Case 13

A 45-year-old woman is admitted to A and E with chest pain. An ECG is performed, which is shown below:

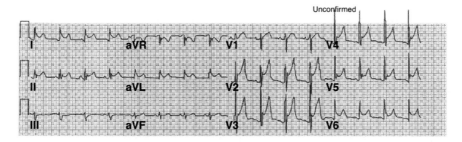

Q. What additional investigations would prove useful?

Q. What management plan would you instigate?

Case 14

A 65-year-old man is admitted as an outpatient for insertion of a pacemaker. Following the procedure he complains of chest pain and shortness of breath. Routine observations demonstrate a pulse rate of 126 beats per minute and a blood pressure of 90/44 mmHg. An ECG is performed, which is shown below:

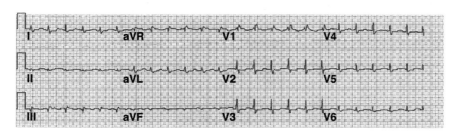

Q. What management plan would you instigate?

Case 15

A 45-year-old woman presents to A and E with shortness of breath. She has a past medical history of ischaemic heart disease and Type II diabetes. She is an occasional drinker and non-smoker. On examination you note minimal bibasal crepitations. A chest X-ray is performed, which is shown below:

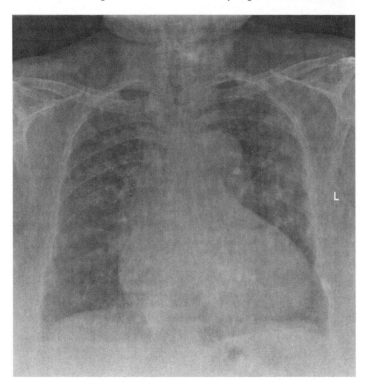

Q. What does the chest X-ray show?

Q. What additional investigations would be useful?

Q. What management plan would you instigate?

2

Endocrinology

Case 1

A 29-year-old man presents to A and E with increasing thirst. He is admitted to hospital for routine investigations, some of which are shown below.

Haemoglobin	12 g/dL
White cell count	13×10^9/L
Platelet count	450×10^9/L
Sodium	149 mmol/L
Potassium	4.1 mmol/L
Urea	9 mmol/L
Creatinine	126 mcmol/L
C-reactive protein	54 mg/L
2-hour plasma glucose	11.6 mmol/L
Fasting plasma glucose	7.2 mmol/L
Anti-GAD antibodies	negative

Q. What management plan would you instigate?

Case 2

You are asked to review a patient's blood results, which are shown below.

Haemoglobin	14 g/dL
White cell count	9 × 10⁹/L
Platelet count	380 × 10⁹/L
Sodium	137 mmol/L
Potassium	4.2 mmol/L
Urea	5 mmol/L
Creatinine	110 mcmol/L
TSH	0.1 mU/L (normal range: 0.5–5.7 mU/L)
T4	62 nmol/L (normal range: 70–140 nmol/L)
T3	0.5 nmol/L (normal range: 1.2–3 nmol/L)

Q. What management plan would you instigate?

Case 3

A 54-year-old man presents to his GP for a routine check-up. Blood tests taken previously demonstrate the following:

Haemoglobin	13 g/dL
White cell count	10 × 10⁹/L
Platelet count	383 × 10⁹/L
Sodium	139 mmol/L
Potassium	4.1 mmol/L
Urea	5 mmol/L
Creatinine	101 mcmol/L
TSH	10.3 mU/L (normal range: 0.5–5.7 mU/L)
T4	79 nmol/L (normal range: 70–140 nmol/L)

Q. What management plan would you instigate?

Case 4

A 54-year-old woman presents to her GP with generalised muscle weakness and bone pain. Up until now she had not visited her GP before. Blood investigations demonstrate the following:

Haemoglobin	12 g/dL
White cell count	9×10^9/L
Platelet count	381×10^9/L
Sodium	135 mmol/L
Potassium	4.5 mmol/L
Urea	15.1 mmol/L
Creatinine	267 mcmol/L
Calcium	2.01 mmol/L (normal range: 2.12–2.65 mmol/L)
Parathyroid hormone	10 pmol/L (normal range: 0.8–8.5 pmol/L)
Creatine kinase	140 U/L (normal range: 25–170 U/L)

Q. What management plan would you instigate?

Case 5

A 64-year-old man presents to A and E with new onset seizures. Blood investigations demonstrate the following:

Haemoglobin	11 g/dL
White cell count	9.5×10^9/L
Platelet count	386×10^9/L
Sodium	133 mmol/L
Potassium	4.1 mmol/L
Urea	10 mmol/L
Creatinine	104 mcmol/L
Calcium	2.01 mmol/L (normal range: 2.12–2.65 mmol/L)
Parathyroid hormone	0.4 pmol/L (normal range: 0.8–8.5 pmol/L)

Q. What management plan would you instigate?

Case 6

A 45-year-old man presents to hospital with increased weight gain and low mood. He is admitted for further tests, the results of which are shown below.

Haemoglobin	14 g/dL
White cell count	11×10^9/L
Platelet count	383×10^9/L
Sodium	134 mmol/L
Potassium	3.9 mmol/L
Urea	10 mmol/L
Creatinine	108 mcmol/L
Serum cortisol post overnight dexamethasone suppression test	4.2 mcg/dL
Late-night salivary cortisol	174 ng/dL

Q. What is the most likely diagnosis?

Case 7

A 54-year-old woman is being reviewed by her GP following initial complaints of feeling tired and weight loss. An array of blood tests were performed, which are shown below.

Haemoglobin	12 g/dL
White cell count	12×10^9/L
Platelet count	386×10^9/L
Sodium	128 mmol/L
Potassium	5.9 mmol/L
Urea	10.2 mmol/L
Creatinine	100 mcmol/L
Serum cortisol post overnight dexamethasone suppression test	1.2 mcg/dL
Late-night salivary cortisol	143 ng/dL
TSH	0.9 mU/L (normal range: 0.5–5.7 mU/L)
T4	85 nmol/L (normal range: 70–140 nmol/L)
Serum cortisol 30 minutes post synacthen	450 nmol/L

Q. What is the most likely diagnosis?

Case 8

A middle-aged woman presents with increasing thirst and urinary frequency. She undergoes the water deprivation test, the results of which are shown below.

Urine osmolality after water deprivation   Urine osmolality after ADH
250 mosmol/kg   250 mosmol/kg

Q. What is the most likely diagnosis?

Case 9

An overweight middle-aged man presents to A and E with increasing thirst. Investigations demonstrate the following:

Haemoglobin	14 g/dL
White cell count	9×10^9/L
Platelet count	280×10^9/L
Sodium	129 mmol/L
Potassium	4.0 mmol/L
Urea	9 mmol/L
Creatinine	151 mcmol/L
Glucose	31 mmol/L
Urine ketones	+++

Arterial blood gas on room air:

pH	7.2
PO_2	10 kPa (normal > 10.6 kPa)
PCO_2	3.8 kPa (normal range: 4.7–6 kPa)
Bicarbonate	12 mmol/L (normal range: 24–30 mmol/L)
Base excess	−3 mmol/L (normal range: −2 to +2 mmol/L)

Q. What management plan would you instigate?

Case 10

A middle-aged woman presents to A and E feeling tired. She has a past medical history of Type II diabetes. Blood investigations demonstrate the following:

Haemoglobin	13 g/dL
White cell count	10×10^9/L
Platelet count	284×10^9/L
Sodium	150 mmol/L
Potassium	5 mmol/L
Urea	9 mmol/L
Creatinine	156 mcmol/L
Glucose	45 mmol/L
Urine ketones	trace

Arterial blood gas on room air:

pH	7.34
PO_2	10 kPa (normal > 10.6 kPa)
PCO_2	5 kPa (normal range: 4.7–6 kPa)
Bicarbonate	22 mmol/L (normal range: 24–30 mmol/L)

Q. What management plan would you instigate?

3

Gastroenterology

Case 1

A 63-year-old gentleman presents to Accident and Emergency (A and E) complaining of abdominal pain and weight loss. On examination you note evidence of jaundice and tenderness in the right upper quadrant. A CT scan is performed and is shown below.

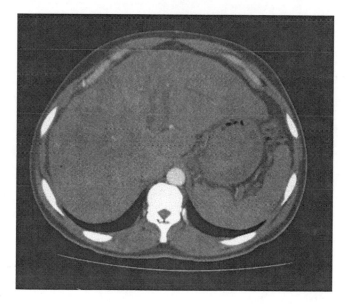

Q. What does the CT scan show?

Q. What additional investigations would be useful?

Q. What management plan would you instigate?

Case 2

A 24-year-old woman presents to A and E with a 1-week history of bloody diarrhoea. She states she has been opening her bowels up to 10 times per day. She also complains of generalised abdominal tenderness. Observations reveal a heart rate of 95 beats per minute, blood pressure of 95/78 mmHg and temperature of 39 °C. Routine blood investigations are as follows:

Haemoglobin	8 g/dL
White cell count	23 × 10⁹/L
Platelet count	500 × 10⁹/L
Sodium	132 mmol/L
Potassium	3 mmol/L
Urea	9 mmol/L
Creatinine	180 mcmol/L
C-reactive protein	156 mg/L

An abdominal X-ray is performed and is shown below.

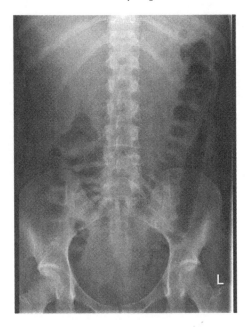

Q. What does the abdominal X-ray show?

Q. What additional investigations would be useful?

Q. What management plan would you instigate?

Case 3

A 35-year-old obese woman presents to A and E with abdominal pain and vomiting. Abdominal examination reveals evidence of generalised abdominal tenderness. A CT abdomen is performed and is shown below.

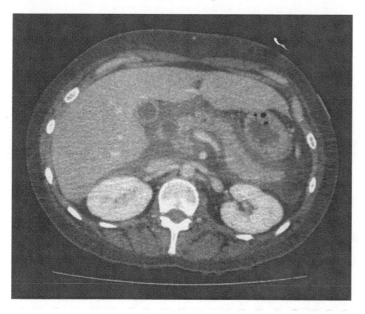

Q. What does the CT show?

Q. What additional investigations would be useful?

Q. What management plan would you instigate?

Case 4

A 37-year-old gentleman presents to A and E with abdominal pain and vomiting. An abdominal X-ray is performed and is shown below.

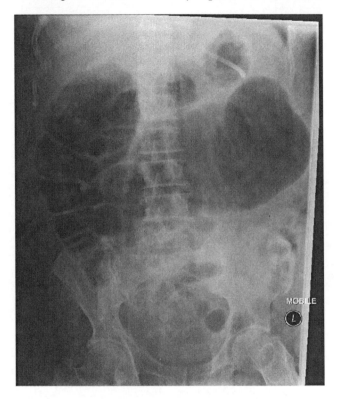

Q. What does the abdominal X-ray show?

Q. What additional investigations would be useful?

Q. What management plan would you instigate?

Case 5

A 51-year-old obese gentleman presents to the gastroenterology outpatients department with central abdominal pain. He is a long-term smoker and occasional drinker. He subsequently undergoes an endoscopy. A section of the histology report is described below.

> *Within the antrum there is evidence of slough and inflammatory debris with neutrophils and active granulation. Upon addition of Giemsa stain, there is a large number of gram negative bacteria adhering to the gastric epithelium, lining the gastric glands as well as mast cells.*

Q. What management plan would you instigate?

Case 6

A 35-year-old woman is admitted to hospital with severe pneumonia. Whilst in hospital she develops diarrhoea. You suggest sending off stool cultures, but your consultant insists on an urgent endoscopy. A section of the histology report is described below.

> *There is evidence of pseudomembranous plaques composed of fibrinous material and polymorphonuclear cells.*

Q. What management plan would you instigate?

Case 7

A 34-year-old alcoholic presents to A and E with vomiting. Blood investigations demonstrate the following:

Haemoglobin	9 g/dL
Platelet count	500 × 10⁹/L
White cell count	18 × 10⁹/L
Sodium	132 mmol/L
Potassium	3.5 mmol/L
Urea	9 mmol/L
Creatinine	149 mcmol/L
C-reactive protein	89 mg/L

Q. What do the above results show?

Q. What management plan would you instigate?

Case 8

A 45-year-old man presents to A and E with new onset confusion. Blood investigations demonstrate the following:

Haemoglobin	10 g/dL
White cell count	21 × 10⁹/L
Platelet count	100 × 10⁹/L
Sodium	130 mmol/L
Potassium	3 mmol/L
Urea	9 mmol/L
Creatinine	170 mcmol/L
Bilirubin	89 mcmol/L (normal range 3–17 mcmol/L)
AST	900 U/L (normal range 5–35 U/L)
ALT	1050 U/L (normal range 5–35 U/L)
INR	2
Glucose	2.6 mmol/L

Q. What do the blood results show?

Q. What additional investigations and management would be useful?

Case 9

A 54-year-old woman presents with weight loss and feeling tired. On examination she is significantly jaundiced. Blood investigations demonstrate the following:

Haemoglobin	12 g/dL
White cell count	15×10^9/L
Platelet count	356×10^9/L
Sodium	134 mmol/L
Potassium	4 mmol/L
Urea	5 mmol/L
Creatinine	122 mcmol/L
Bilirubin	68 mcmol/L (normal range: 3–17 mcmol/L)
ALT	300 U/L (normal range: 5–35 U/L)
AST	256 U/L (normal range: 5–35 U/L)
ALP	140 U/L (normal range: 30–150 U/L)
IgG	positive
ANA	positive
Anti-smooth muscle antibodies	positive

Q. What do the above results show?

Q. What additional investigations would be useful?

Q. What management plan would you instigate?

Case 10

A 45-year-old gentleman presents with increased stool frequency and abdominal pain. He undergoes an endoscopy. A section of the histology report is described below.

There is evidence of transmural infiltration with neutrophils and lymphocytes with skip lesions and granulomas.

Q. What management plan would you instigate?

Case 11

A 25-year-old woman presents with abdominal bloating and loose stools. Blood investigations demonstrate the following:

Haemoglobin	9 g/dL
White cell count	12 × 10⁹/L
Platelet count	400 × 10⁹/L
Sodium	134 mmol/L
Potassium	4 mmol/L
Urea	6 mmol/L
Creatinine	149 mcmol/L
Calcium	1.97 mmol/L
Magnesium	1.1 mmol/L
Albumin	29 g/L
PT	30 seconds (normal range: 10–14 seconds)

Q. What additional investigations may be useful?

Case 12

A 35-year-old man is referred to the gastroenterology outpatient clinic as his GP was concerned about the possibility of hepatitis infection. You review the results of some of his investigations, which are shown below.

HBsAg	positive
Anti-HBs	negative
HBeAg	positive
Anti-HBe	negative
Anti-HBc	positive
IgM anti-HBc	positive
HBV DNA	positive
ALT	154 U/L

Q. What management plan would you instigate?

4

Neurology

Case 1

A 45-year-old man presents to Accident and Emergency (A and E) with sudden onset left-sided weakness and a headache. A CT head is performed which is shown below.

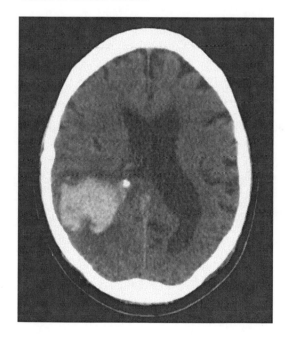

Q. What does the CT show?

Q. What management plan would you instigate?

Case 2

A 25-year-old woman presents to A and E with new onset sensory loss and muscle cramps. She undergoes a MRI brain and lumbar puncture, the results of which are shown below.

Appearance	clear and colourless
Gram stain	negative
Red blood cells	nil
Lymphocytes	4/mm³ (normal < 5/mm³)
Polymorphs	nil
Protein	18 g/L (normal < 0.4 g/L)
Glucose	6 mmol/L (normal > 2.2 mmol/L)
Opening pressure	150 mm (normal < 200 mm)
Oligoclonal bands	positive

Q. What management plan would you instigate?

Case 3

A 58-year-old woman is being followed up in a neurology outpatient clinic. She complains of muscle fatigue and underwent repetitive nerve stimulation of a weak muscle, the results of which are illustrated below.

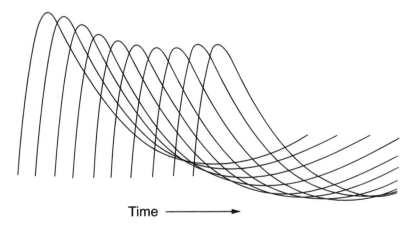

Time ——————→

Q. What management plan would you instigate?

Case 4

An 18-year-old girl presents to A and E with neck stiffness and a rash. A CT head is performed and later a lumbar puncture, the results of which are shown below.

Red blood cells	nil
Polymorphs	85%
Protein	1 g/L (normal < 0.4 g/L)
Glucose	1.5 mmol/L (normal > 2.2 mmol/L)
Opening pressure	350 mm (normal < 200 mm)

Q. What management plan would you instigate?

Case 5

A 30-year-old woman presents to A and E. Her friend who is accompanying her comments that she has been acting strangely over the past few days and doesn't seem her usual self. A CT head is performed and a lumbar puncture, the results of which are shown below.

Red blood cells	nil
Lymphocytes	65/mm^3 (normal < 5/mm^3)
Polymorphs	nil
Protein	6 g/L (normal: 0.4 g/L)
Glucose	3 mmol/L (normal > 2.2 mmol/L)

Q. What management plan would you instigate?

5

Overdose

Case 1

A 27-year-old woman presents to Accident and Emergency (A and E) with vomiting and hearing disturbance. She has a medical history of depression. An arterial blood gas on room air demonstrates the following:

pH	7.55
PO_2	10 kPa (normal > 10.6 kPa)
PCO_2	3.4 kPa (normal range: 4.7–6 kPa)
Bicarbonate	26 mmol/L (normal range: 24–30 mmol/L)
Base excess	–1.5 mmol/L (normal range: –2 to +2 mmol/L)

The blood gas is repeated some time later and demonstrates the following:

pH	7.24
PO_2	10 kPa
PCO_2	5 kPa
Bicarbonate	18 mmol/L
Base excess	–3 mmol/L

Q. What management plan would you instigate?

Case 2

A 34-year-old woman with a history of depression presents to A and E following an overdose. She refuses to tell you what she has taken but is willing to have blood tests, the results of which are shown below.

Haemoglobin	16 g/dL
White cell count	8×10^9/L
Platelet count	354×10^9/L
Sodium	136 mmol/L
Potassium	4.1 mmol/L
Urea	9 mmol/L
Creatinine	200 mcmol/L
Bilirubin	14 mcmol/L (normal range: 3–17 mcmol/L)
ALT	189 U/L (normal range: 5–35 U/L)
AST	200 U/L (normal range: 5–35 U/L)
ALP	89 U/L (normal range: 30–150 U/L)
INR	2.5

Q. What management plan would you instigate?

6

Renal

Case 1

A 35-year-old gentleman presents to Accident and Emergency (A and E) with haematuria. A renal ultrasound proves unremarkable and he is referred for a renal biopsy. A few hours post procedure he complains of pain over the biopsy site. Abdominal examination reveals tenderness over the right flank. Routine observations demonstrate a blood pressure of 90/55 mmHg and a pulse rate of 120 beats per minute. He undergoes an urgent CT scan.

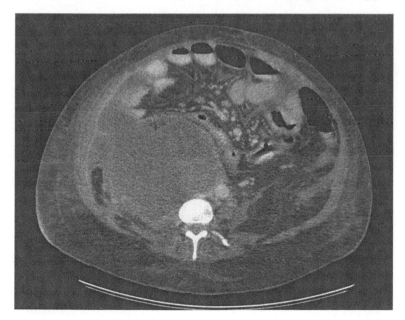

Q. What does the CT show?

Case 2

A 45-year-old woman presents to A and E with abdominal pain. She also complains of difficulty in passing urine. Routine blood investigations demonstrate the following:

Haemoglobin	12 g/dL
Platelet count	250×10^9/L
White cell count	11×10^9/L
Sodium	137 mmol/L
Potassium	6 mmol/L
Urea	9 mmol/L
Creatinine	225 mcmol/L

Three months ago, a blood test by her GP indicated a potassium of 4.5 mmol/L, urea of 6 mmol/L and creatinine of 150 mcmol/L.

Q. What do the latest blood results show?

Q. What additional investigations may be useful?

Q. What management plan would you instigate?

Case 3

A 35-year-old woman presented to A and E with increased facial swelling.
Blood investigations demonstrated the following:

Haemoglobin	12 g/dL
White cell count	7×10^9/L
Platelet count	400×10^9/L
Sodium	135 mmol/L
Potassium	5 mmol/L
Urea	6.5 mmol/L
Creatinine	189 mcmol/L
Albumin	20 g/L

Urinalysis demonstrated:

Protein	2+
Leucocytes	trace
Nitrites	trace
Blood	trace

Q. What additional investigations may be useful?

Q. What management plan would you instigate?

Case 4

A 65-year-old man presents to his GP. He complains of a new onset itch and feeling tired. Blood investigations demonstrate the following:

Haemoglobin	8 g/dL
MCV	85 fL (normal range: 76–96 fL)
White cell count	10×10^9/L
Platelet count	350×10^9/L
Sodium	135 mmol/L
Potassium	4.2 mmol/L
Urea	10 mmol/L
Creatinine	250 mcmol/L
Calcium	1.97 mmol/L
eGFR	27 mL/min/1.73 m^2

Q. What management plan would you instigate?

Case 5

A 15-year-old boy presents to A and E with new onset diarrhoea. He had recently visited an amusement park and felt unwell after eating a hamburger. Blood investigations demonstrate:

Haemoglobin	9 g/dL
White cell count	15×10^9/L
Platelet count	100×10^9/L
Sodium	140 mmol/L
Potassium	5.1 mmol/L
Urea	10 mmol/L
Creatinine	180 mcmol/L
C-reactive protein	180 mg/L
PT	11 seconds (normal range: 10–14 seconds)
APTT	37 seconds (normal range: 35–45 seconds)
INR	<1
Blood film	helmet-shaped cells noted

Q. What management plan would you instigate?

Case 6

A 54-year-old man presents to A and E with worsening shortness of breath. He has a past medical history of lung cancer diagnosed 6 weeks ago. Investigations demonstrate the following:

Haemoglobin	12 g/dL
White cell count	11×10^9/L
Platelet count	400×10^9/L
Sodium	124 mmol/L
Potassium	4 mmol/L
Urea	7 mmol/L
Creatinine	149 mcmol/L
Urine sodium	25 mmol/L
Urine osmolality	560 mosmol/kg
Plasma osmolality	210 mosmol/kg

Q. What management plan would you instigate?

Case 7

A 45-year-old woman presents to hospital with abdominal pain and reduced urinary frequency. Bloods are taken and a routine ECG is performed, as demonstrated below.

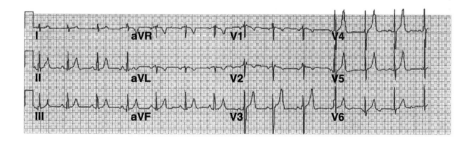

Q. What management plan would you instigate in view of this ECG?

Case 8

A 65-year-old man presents to his GP following routine blood investigations, which are shown below. He has no past medical history, but family history reveals his sister had a myocardial infarction at age 58. On examination you note yellow-coloured lesions on the extensor tendons of his hands.

Haemoglobin	13 g/dL
White cell count	7×10^9/L
Platelet count	201×10^9/L
Sodium	139 mmol/L
Potassium	4.5 mmol/L
Urea	5 mmol/L
Creatinine	110 mcmol/L
Total cholesterol	10.2 mmol/L
LDL cholesterol	6.4 mmol/L

Q. What management plan would you instigate?

Case 9

A 54-year-old alcoholic is admitted to hospital with severe onset abdominal pain. A CT scan demonstrates evidence of acute pancreatitis. A routine ECG is performed and is shown below.

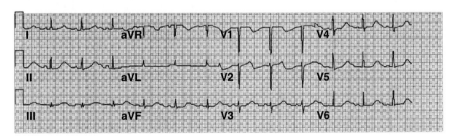

Q. What management plan would you instigate in view of this ECG?

7

Haematology

Case 1

A 32-year-old woman presents to her GP for a review of her blood results, which are shown below.

Haemoglobin	8.4 g/dL
White cell count	10×10^9/L
MCV	72 fL (normal range: 76–96 fL)
MCH	23 pg (normal range: 27–32 pg)
Platelet count	200×10^9/L
Sodium	137 mmol/L
Potassium	4.2 mmol/L
Urea	6 mmol/L
Creatinine	135 mcmol/L
Ferritin	4 mcg/L (normal range: 12–200 mcg/L)

Q. What additional investigations would be useful?

Q. What management plan would you instigate?

Case 2

You are asked to review the following blood results for a patient who presented to the outpatient clinic.

Haemoglobin	9 g/dL
White cell count	5 × 10⁹/L
Platelet count	179 × 10⁹/L
MCV	72 fL (normal range: 76–96 fL)
MCH	30 pg (normal range: 27–32 pg)
Sodium	140 mmol/L
Potassium	4.7 mmol/L
Urea	6 mmol/L
Creatinine	101 mcmol/L
Ferritin	300 mcg/L (normal range: 12–200 mcg/L)
Blood film	evidence of basophilic stippling

Q. What management plan would you instigate?

Case 3

You are asked to review a patient who has presented with chest pain and blurring of vision. On examination you note evidence of significant erythroderma. Blood investigations demonstrate the following:

Haemoglobin	14 g/dL
White cell count	41 × 10⁹/L
Platelet count	550 × 10⁹/L
Neutrophils	19 × 10⁹/L (normal range: 2–7.5 × 10⁹/L)
Eosinophils	2.1 × 10⁹/L (normal range: 0.04–0.44 × 10⁹/L)
Sodium	140 mmol/L
Potassium	4.1 mmol/L
Urea	7 mmol/L
Creatinine	149 mcmol/L

Q. What management plan would you instigate?

Case 4

You are reviewing a patient who has presented to the outpatient department with shortness of breath. Blood investigations demonstrate the following:

Haemoglobin	8.4 g/dL
White cell count	4.5×10^9/L
MCV	105 fL (normal range: 76–96 fL)
MCH	42 pg (normal range: 27–32 pg)
Platelet count	155×10^9/L
Sodium	134 mmol/L
Potassium	4.5 mmol/L
Urea	6.5 mmol/L
Creatinine	148 mcmol/L

Urinary measurement of radiolabelled B_{12} without intrinsic factor – low
Urinary measurement of radiolabelled B_{12} with intrinsic factor – normal

Q. What management plan would you instigate?

Case 5

A 45-year-old woman presents with chest pain. Blood investigations demonstrate the following:

Haemoglobin	8.4 g/dL
MCV	105 fL (normal range: 76–96 fL)
Platelet count	250×10^9/L
White cell count	8×10^9/L
Sodium	134 mmol/L
Potassium	4.3 mmol/L
Urea	6.4 mmol/L
Creatinine	145 mcmol/L
Bilirubin	65 mcmol/L (normal range: 3–17 mcmol/L)
AST	34 U/L (normal range: 5–35 U/L)
ALT	33 U/L (normal range: 5–35 U/L)
ALP	110 U/L (normal range: 30–150 U/L)
LDH	320 U/L (normal range: 70–250 U/L)

Q. What management plan would you instigate?

Case 6

A 32-year-old man presents to Accident and Emergency (A and E) with sudden onset pain in his arms and legs. Blood investigations demonstrate the following:

Haemoglobin	7 g/dL
Reticulocyte count	150 × 10⁹/L (normal range: 25–100 × 10⁹/L)
White cell count	21 × 10⁹/L
Platelet count	550 × 10⁹/L
Sodium	140 mmol/L
Potassium	3.5 mmol/L
Urea	8 mmol/L
Creatinine	140 mcmol/L
Bilirubin	78 mcmol/L (normal range: 3–17 mcmol/L)
ALT	33 U/L (normal range: 5–35 U/L)
AST	34 U/L (normal range: 5–35 U/L)
ALP	140 U/L (normal range: 30–150 U/L)
Blood film	target cells

Q. What additional investigations would be useful?

Q. What management plan would you instigate?

Case 7

An 8-year-old boy presents to his GP for a routine blood test following a flu-like illness. Blood investigations demonstrate the following:

Haemoglobin	14 g/dL
Platelet count	15×10^9/L
White cell count	10×10^9/L
Sodium	134 mmol/L
Potassium	4.2 mmol/L
Urea	6 mmol/L
Creatinine	140 mcmol/L

Q. What management plan would you instigate?

Case 8

A 20-year-old man presents to A and E with muscle weakness. Routine blood investigations demonstrate the following:

Haemoglobin	9 g/dL
White cell count	12×10^9/L
Platelet count	200×10^9/L
Sodium	134 mmol/L
Potassium	4.2 mmol/L
Urea	6.1 mmol/L
Creatinine	150 mmol/L
INR	<1
Prothrombin time	11 seconds (normal range: 10–14 seconds)
APTT	54 seconds (normal range: 35–45 seconds)

Q. What management plan would you instigate?

Case 9

A middle-aged man presents with widespread bruising. Blood investigations demonstrate the following:

Haemoglobin	9.4 g/dL
White cell count	11×10^9/L
Platelet count	250×10^9/L
Sodium	134 mmol/L
Potassium	4.2 mmol/L
Urea	6.1 mmol/L
Creatinine	130 mcmol/L
INR	<1
Prothrombin time	12 seconds (normal range: 10–14 seconds)
APTT	58 seconds (normal range: 35–45 seconds)
Bleeding time	+++

Q. What management plan would you instigate?

Case 10

A 54-year-old woman presents to A and E feeling generally unwell after receiving her third cycle of chemotherapy. On examination you note a temperature of 38 °C. Blood investigations demonstrate the following:

Haemoglobin	14 g/dL
White cell count	19×10^9/L
Neutrophils	0.8×10^9/L (normal range: $2–7.5 \times 10^9$/L)
Lymphocytes	1.5×10^9/L (normal range: $1.3–3.5 \times 10^9$/L)
Eosinophils	0.34×10^9/L (normal range: $0.04–0.44 \times 10^9$/L)
Platelet count	260×10^9/L
Sodium	135 mmol/L
Potassium	3.7 mmol/L
Urea	5.4 mmol/L
Creatinine	147 mcmol/L
C-reactive protein	150 mg/L

Q. What management plan would you instigate?

Case 11

You are reviewing the blood results of a patient admitted with acute pancreatitis, which are shown below:

Haemoglobin	9.5 g/dL
White cell count	15×10^9/L
Platelet count	49×10^9/L
Sodium	134 mmol/L
Potassium	3.9 mmol/L
Urea	5.9 mmol/L
Creatinine	147 mcmol/L
D-dimer	2.5 mg/L (normal < 0.5 mg/L)
Prothrombin time	21 seconds (normal range: 10–14 seconds)
Fibrinogen level	0.8 g/L (normal range: 1.5–3 g/L)

Q. What management plan would you instigate?

Case 12

A middle-aged man presents to hospital with increasing fatigue. Blood investigations and a subsequent bone marrow aspirate demonstrate the following:

Haemoglobin	8.6 g/dL
White cell count	53×10^9/L
Platelet count	109×10^9/L
Sodium	134 mmol/L
Potassium	3.9 mmol/L
Urea	5.6 mmol/L
Creatinine	117 mcmol/L
Bone marrow aspirate	Blast cells +++

Q. What management plan would you instigate?

Case 13

An elderly gentleman presents to A and E complaining of neck swelling. Routine blood investigations demonstrate the following:

Haemoglobin	9.4 g/dL
White cell count	25×10^9/L
Neutrophils	6.5×10^9/L (normal range: $2-7.5 \times 10^9$/L)
Eosinophils	0.34×10^9/L (normal range: $0.04-0.44 \times 10^9$/L)
Lymphocytes	6×10^9/L (normal range: $1.3-3.5 \times 10^9$/L)
Platelet count	450×10^9/L
Sodium	134 mmol/L
Potassium	3.9 mmol/L
Urea	5.6 mmol/L
Creatinine	140 mcmol/L
Blood film	presence of smudge cells noted

Q. What management plan would you instigate?

Case 14

A 45-year-old man presents to A and E with blurring of vision. Abdominal examination demonstrates evidence of splenomegaly. Blood investigations demonstrate the following:

Haemoglobin	19 g/dL
MCV	80 fL (normal range: 76–96 fL)
Haematocrit	0.8 l/L (normal range: 0.4–0.54 l/L)
White cell count	17×10^9/L
Neutrophil count	15×10^9/L (normal range: $2-7.5 \times 10^9$/L)
Platelet count	550×10^9/L
Sodium	134 mmol/L
Potassium	4.2 mmol/L
Urea	5.8 mmol/L
Creatinine	145 mcmol/L

Q. What management plan would you instigate?

Case 15

An elderly woman presents to hospital with weight loss and night sweats. Blood investigations demonstrate the following:

Haemoglobin	9 g/dL
White cell count	21×10^9/L
Platelet count	560×10^9/L
Sodium	137 mmol/L
Potassium	4.1 mmol/L
Urea	5.8 mmol/L
Creatinine	114 mcmol/L
Blood film	teardrop-shaped red cells

Q. What management plan would you instigate?

Case 16

A 54-year-old man is referred to the haematology outpatients department with non-specific bone pain. Investigations demonstrate the following:

Haemoglobin	9.1 g/dL
MCV	85 fL (normal range: 76–96 fL)
White cell count	8×10^9/L
Platelet count	450×10^9/L
Sodium	134 mmol/L
Potassium	4.3 mmol/L
Calcium	3.1 mmol/L
Urea	9.1 mmol/L
Creatinine	180 mcmol/L
Serum electrophoresis	M-protein 35 g/L

Q. What management plan would you instigate?

8

Rheumatology

Case 1

A 64-year-old woman presents to her GP with pain in several of her small hand joints for more than 8 weeks. Blood investigations demonstrate the following:

Haemoglobin	8.1 g/dL
White cell count	14×10^9/L
Platelet count	560×10^9/L
Sodium	134 mmol/L
Potassium	4.1 mmol/L
Urea	5.4 mmol/L
Creatinine	140 mcmol/L
C-reactive protein	120 mg/L
Rheumatoid factor	negative
Anti-citrullinated protein antibody (ACPA)	positive

Q. What management plan would you instigate?

Case 2

A 23-year-old man presents to Accident and Emergency (A and E) with a swollen knee joint. Joint aspiration confirms the following:

Appearance	yellow turbid
Neutrophil count	>95%
White cell count	95 000/mm^3 (normal < 200 mm^3)
Gram stain	Gram-positive cocci

Q. What additional investigations would be useful?

Case 3

A 43-year-old man presents to A and E with a swollen and tender toe. Investigations demonstrate the following:

Haemoglobin	13.2 g/dL
White cell count	15 × 10^9/L
Platelet count	512 × 10^9/L
Sodium	142 mmol/L
Potassium	4.2 mmol/L
Urea	6.1 mmol/L
Creatinine	134 mcmol/L
Serum urate	116 mcmol/L (normal range: 110–420 mcmol/L)
Joint aspirate	negatively birefringent urate crystals

Q. What management plan would you instigate?

Case 4

A 35-year-old woman presents with joint pain, mouth ulcers and a facial rash. Blood investigations demonstrate the following:

Haemoglobin	7 g/dL
White cell count	2.7×10^9/L
Platelet count	100×10^9/L
Sodium	133 mmol/L
Potassium	4.1 mmol/L
Urea	6.5 mmol/L
Creatinine	189 mcmol/L
ANA	positive
Anti-cyclic citrullinated peptide antibody (anti-CCP)	negative
Rheumatoid factor	negative
Anti-histone antibody	negative
Anti-Ro antibody	negative
Anti-La antibody	negative
Anti-centromere antibody	negative
Anti-Scl-70 antibody	negative
Anti-Jo-1 antibody	negative

Q. What management plan would you instigate?

Case 5

A 39-year-old woman presents with difficulty in swallowing and discolouration of her fingers and toes. Blood investigations demonstrate the following:

Haemoglobin	9 g/dL
White cell count	10×10^9/L
Platelet count	124×10^9/L
Sodium	134 mmol/L
Potassium	4.2 mmol/L
Urea	6 mmol/L
Creatinine	110 mcmol/L
ANA	negative
Anti-CCP	negative
Rheumatoid factor	negative
Anti-histone antibody	negative
Anti-Ro antibody	negative
Anti-La antibody	negative
Anti-centromere antibody	positive
Anti-Scl-70 antibody	positive
Anti-Jo-1 antibody	negative

Q. What management plan would you instigate?

Case 6

A 47-year-old woman is seen in the rheumatology outpatient department with new onset muscle weakness and a rash. Blood investigations demonstrate the following:

Haemoglobin	15 g/dL
White cell count	10×10^9/L
Platelet count	179×10^9/L
Sodium	134 mmol/L
Potassium	4.2 mmol/L
Urea	6 mmol/L
Creatinine	115 mcmol/L
ANA	negative
Anti-CCP	negative
Rheumatoid factor	negative
Anti-histone antibody	negative
Anti-Ro antibody	negative
Anti-La antibody	negative
Anti-centromere antibody	negative
Anti-Scl-70 antibody	negative
Anti-Jo-1 antibody	negative
Anti-Mi-2 antibody	positive

Q. What management plan would you instigate?

Case 7

A 63-year-old man presents with haemoptysis and joint discomfort. Blood investigations demonstrate the following:

Haemoglobin	11 g/dL
White cell count	23×10^9/L
Platelet count	550×10^9/L
Sodium	134 mmol/L
Potassium	4.2 mmol/L
Urea	15 mmol/L
Creatinine	214 mcmol/L
C-reactive protein	215 mg/L
ANA	negative
Anti-CCP	negative
Rheumatoid factor	negative
Anti-histone antibody	negative
Anti-Ro antibody	negative
Anti-La antibody	negative
Anti-centromere antibody	negative
Anti-Scl-70 antibody	negative
Anti-Jo-1 antibody	negative
Anti-Mi-2 antibody	negative
PR3 ANCA	positive

Q. What management plan would you instigate?

Respiratory

Case 1

A 35-year-old intravenous drug abuser presents with shortness of breath and a dry cough over a 1-week period. In addition he states he has been feeling feverish and experiencing generalised muscle weakness. Routine observations demonstrate a heart rate of 125 beats per minute, blood pressure of 98/75 mmHg and oxygen saturations of 89% on room air. Chest auscultation demonstrates crepitations at the left base. A chest X-ray is performed and is shown below.

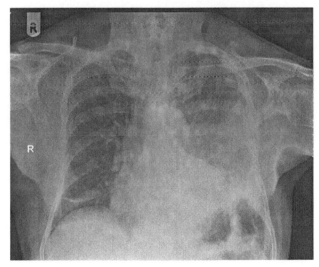

Q. What does the chest X-ray show?

Q. What additional investigations would be useful?

Q. What management plan would you instigate?

Case 2

A 42-year-old Bangladeshi gentleman presents to Accident and Emergency (A and E) complaining of sudden onset shortness of breath. On further questioning, he states he has been experiencing a cough productive of blood-tinged sputum. A chest X-ray is ordered, which is shown below.

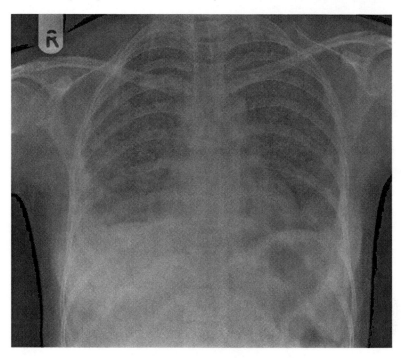

Q. What does the chest X-ray show?

Q. What additional investigations would be useful?

Q. What management plan would you instigate?

Case 3

A 65-year-old man presents with a dry cough and breathlessness on exertion. He recently went to see his GP who prescribed a course of amoxicillin. Despite completing a 7-day course he comments his cough progressively got worse and he 'can't seem to shift it'. He has a past medical history of Type II diabetes and is currently taking metformin. He is a non-smoker and drinks alcohol on occasion. Routine observations demonstrate an oxygen saturation of 94% on room air. A chest X-ray is ordered which is shown below.

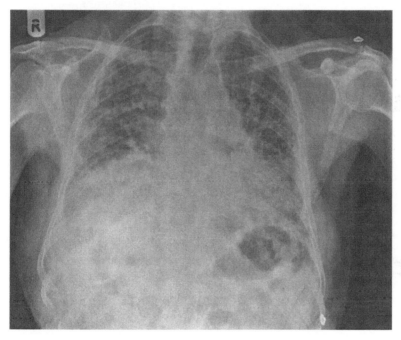

Q. What does the chest X-ray show?

Q. What additional investigations would be useful?

Q. What management plan would you instigate?

Case 4

A 67-year-old gentleman presented to A and E with a dry cough and shortness of breath. He had smoked all his life, having tried to cut down previously. His mother had died at the age of 50 from lung cancer and his father was suffering from angina. Routine observations demonstrated an oxygen saturation of 88% on room air. Chest auscultation demonstrated evidence of a wheeze bilaterally on expiration. A chest X-ray was performed and is shown below.

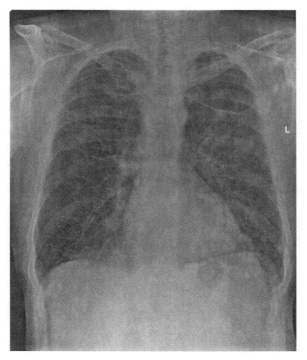

Q. What does the chest X-ray show?

Q. What additional investigations would be useful?

Q. What management plan would you instigate?

Case 5

A 19-year-old male presents to A and E with sudden onset chest pain and shortness of breath. He describes his pain as sharp and stabbing in nature, being particularly worse on inspiration. He went to see his GP earlier, who prescribed paracetamol. Routine observations demonstrate an oxygen saturation of 90% on room air. A chest X-ray is ordered and is shown below.

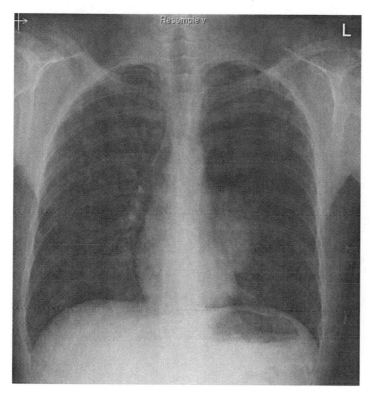

Q. What does the chest X-ray show?

Q. What additional investigations would be useful?

Q. What management plan would you instigate?

Case 6

A 61-year-old farmer presented to A and E with shortness of breath. He described finding it difficult to breathe about 6 hours after finishing work that day. In addition to this he described a tight feeling in his chest as well as generalised muscle weakness. On examination you noted subtle crepitations bilaterally but no wheeze. Cardiovascular, abdominal and neurological examination proved unremarkable. A chest X-ray is performed and is shown below.

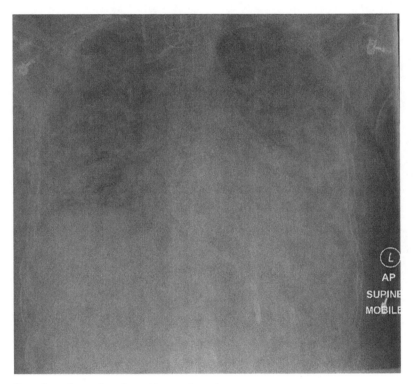

Q. What does the chest X-ray show?

Q. What additional investigations would be useful?

Q. What management plan would you instigate?

Case 7

A 55-year-old woman presents to A and E with a 3-week history of grad-ual shortness of breath. During the consultation she admits to coughing up blood on occasion. She is a lifelong smoker and occasional drinker. On examination you note evidence of finger clubbing. A chest X-ray is ordered and is shown below.

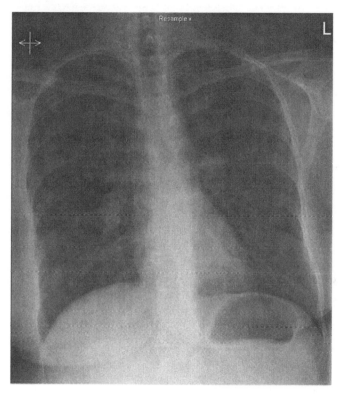

Q. What does the chest X-ray show?

Q. What additional investigations would be useful?

Q. What management plan would you instigate?

Case 8

A 25-year-old woman presents to A and E with shortness of breath. She comments her breathing is particularly worse at night and first thing in the morning. She has no past medical history and is on no current medication. Routine observations demonstrate a heart rate of 130 beats per minute, blood pressure of 110/60 mmHg, respiratory rate of 35 breaths per minute and oxygen saturations of 90% on room air. On examination you note evidence of a wheeze bilaterally but no crepitations. An arterial blood gas is taken on room air and is shown below.

pH	7.55
PO_2	8 kPa (normal > 10.6 kPa)
PCO_2	3.2 kPa (normal range: 4.7–6 kPa)
Bicarbonate	23 mmol/L (normal range: 24–30 mmol/L)
Base excess	+1 mmol/L (normal range: −2 to +2 mmol/L)

Q. What does the arterial blood gas show?

Q. What additional investigations would be useful?

Q. What management plan would you instigate?

Case 9

A 43-year-old man presents to A and E with chest pain and shortness of breath. He is a lifelong smoker and recently flew to Australia to see his sister. Routine observations reveal an oxygen saturation of 89% on room air. An ECG taken on arrival is shown below.

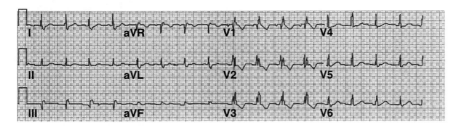

Q. What does the ECG show?

Q. What additional investigations would be useful?

Q. What management plan would you instigate?

Answers

1 Cardiology

Case 1

The ECG demonstrates evidence of sinus tachycardia. In accordance with the UK Resuscitation Council, sinus tachycardia is best managed according to the following algorithm:

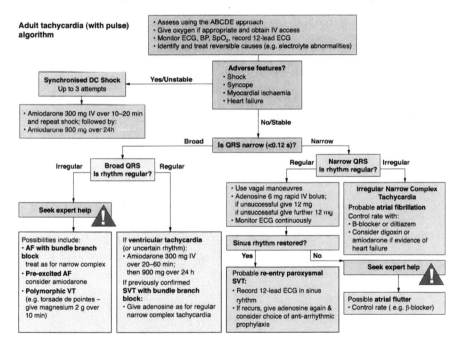

FIGURE 1.1 Tachycardia. Reproduced with the kind permission of the Resuscitation Council (UK).

Case 2

The ECG demonstrates sinus bradycardia. In accordance with the UK Resuscitation Council, the management of bradycardia is as follows:

Adult bradycardia algorithm

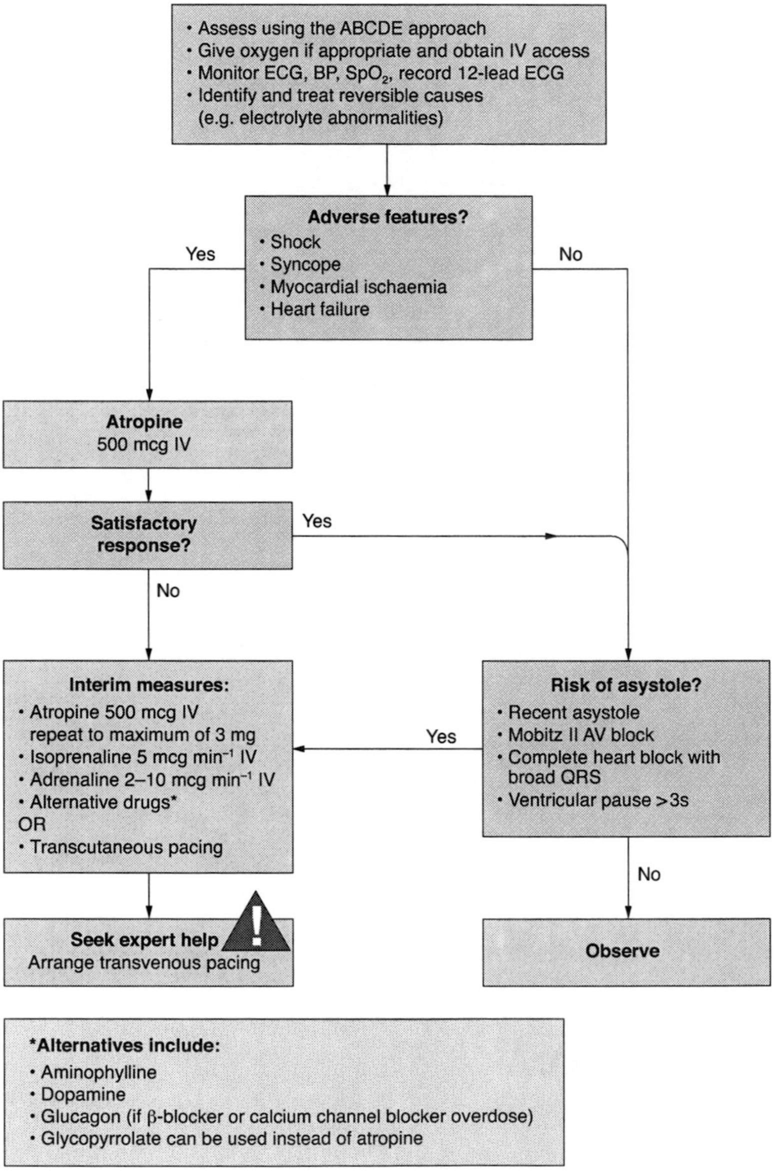

- Assess using the ABCDE approach
- Give oxygen if appropriate and obtain IV access
- Monitor ECG, BP, SpO₂, record 12-lead ECG
- Identify and treat reversible causes
  (e.g. electrolyte abnormalities)

Adverse features?
- Shock
- Syncope
- Myocardial ischaemia
- Heart failure

Yes

No

Atropine
500 mcg IV

Satisfactory response?

Yes

No

Interim measures:
- Atropine 500 mcg IV
  repeat to maximum of 3 mg
- Isoprenaline 5 mcg min⁻¹ IV
- Adrenaline 2–10 mcg min⁻¹ IV
- Alternative drugs*
OR
- Transcutaneous pacing

Yes

Risk of asystole?
- Recent asystole
- Mobitz II AV block
- Complete heart block with
  broad QRS
- Ventricular pause >3s

No

Seek expert help
Arrange transvenous pacing

Observe

*Alternatives include:
- Aminophylline
- Dopamine
- Glucagon (if β-blocker or calcium channel blocker overdose)
- Glycopyrrolate can be used instead of atropine

FIGURE 1.2 Bradycardia. Reproduced with the kind permission of the Resuscitation Council (UK).

Case 3

The ECG demonstrates evidence of atrial fibrillation (AF). In accordance with NICE guidelines, once a diagnosis of AF is confirmed, patients should be stratified according to the risk of stroke/thromboembolism.

Risk	Features	Management
High	Previous ischaemic stroke/TIA or thromboembolic event Age ≥75 with hypertension, diabetes or vascular disease Clinical evidence of valve disease or heart failure, or impaired LV function on echocardiography	Anticoagulation with warfarin. Target INR 2.5 If contraindicated treat with aspirin
Moderate	Age ≥65 with no high risk factors Age <75 with hypertension, diabetes or vascular disease	Consider anticoagulation or aspirin
Low	Age <65 with no moderate or high risk factors	Aspirin 75–300 mg/day if no contraindications

The management of AF then relies upon controlling rate or rhythm.

Rhythm control applies to those:
- who are symptomatic
- who are younger
- presenting for the first time with lone AF
- who have developed AF secondary to a treated or corrected precipitant
- with congestive heart failure.

Rate control applies to those:
- who are over 65
- with coronary artery disease
- with contraindications to antiarrhythmic drugs
- unsuitable for cardioversion.

Rhythm control relies upon the use of beta blockers or amiodarone. Rate control relies primarily on beta blockers, calcium channel blockers or digoxin.

Case 4

The ECG demonstrates evidence of first-degree heart block in view of the prolonged PR interval. In general no intervention is required in these cases if the patient is asymptomatic. However, in this case the patient's beta blocker should be stopped and in severe cases a pacemaker may prove beneficial.

Case 5

The ECG demonstrates evidence of complete heart block. Such cases are best managed with atropine or transcutaneous pacing.

Case 6

The ECG demonstrates evidence of an inferior posterior MI (note ST elevation in leads II, III and AVF (inferior) and tall R waves with ST depression in leads V1–V3. In cases of an ST elevation MI, SIGN guidelines recommend 300 mg of aspirin and 300 mg of clopidogrel in addition to low molecular weight heparin or fondaparinux. Oral beta blockers should be commenced if patients are not significantly hypotensive. Glycaemic control is essential in those with a serum glucose >11.1 mmol/L. Patients with ST elevation should be treated immediately with primary PCI. Such patients should also be treated with a glycoprotein IIb/IIIa receptor antagonist. When PCI cannot be offered within 90 minutes of diagnosis, patients should receive thrombolytic therapy. All patients should be commenced on long-term statins and ACE inhibitors.

Case 7

In view of the history and ECG, this patient is demonstrating evidence of digoxin toxicity. Visual disturbances in the form of yellow-green haloes are particularly common. The ECG demonstrates the classic reversed tick of the ST segment. Digibind is a useful agent for reversing digoxin toxicity and is utilised in cases of arrhythmias and haemodynamic instability, hyperkalaemia and disturbances in mental status.

Case 8

The ECG demonstrates evidence of left bundle branch block (LBBB). Causes of LBBB include myocardial infarction, hypertension, cardiomyopathy and myocarditis.

Case 9
The ECG demonstrates evidence of left ventricular hypertrophy secondary to hypertension. It is generally accepted that hypertension is defined as a blood pressure greater than 140/90 mmHg after separate measurements.

The management of hypertension as per NICE is age and ethnicity dependent. Those under the age of 55 are started on an ACE inhibitor, whereas those over the age of 55 or people of African or Caribbean origin should be commenced on a calcium channel blocker. If this fails to be of benefit, ACE inhibitors are used in combination with calcium channel blockers followed by the addition of a thiazide-like diuretic, alpha blocker or beta blocker.

Case 10
The ECG demonstrates VT. In accordance with the UK Resuscitation Council, the management in Figure 1.3 should be instigated (*see* p. 68).

Case 11
The ECG demonstrates evidence of atrial flutter. Management of atrial flutter involves the use of medical treatment in the form of beta blockers, calcium channel blockers or flecanide, as well as radiofrequency ablation.

Case 12
The ECG demonstrates evidence of Wolff–Parkinson–White (WPW) syndrome (note the short PR interval and slurred upstroke of the QRS). The management of WPW syndrome relies primarily on the use of radiofrequency ablation.

Case 13
The ECG demonstrates evidence of concave ST segment elevation in keeping with a diagnosis of pericarditis. In accordance with the European Society of Cardiology (ESC), patients with suspected pericarditis should have blood investigations including an ESR, CRP, LDH, white cell count and troponin. A chest X-ray and ECHO are also recommended. In cases of tamponade or effusion, additional investigations include pericardiocentesis and drainage, CT, MRI or pericardioscopy and biopsy.

The mainstay form of treatment as per the ESC is NSAIDs. Colchicine is also an effective agent.

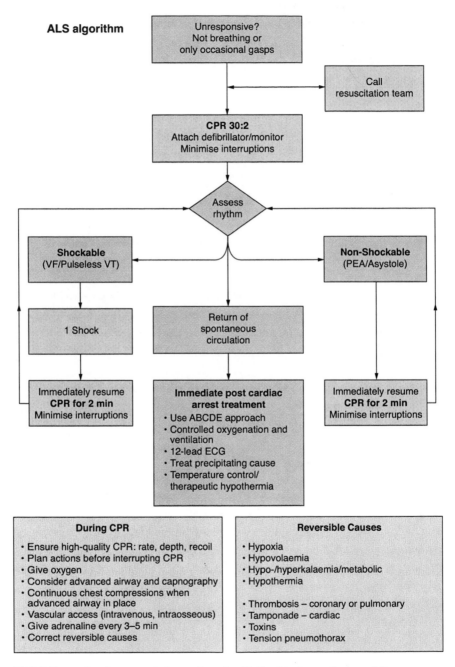

ALS algorithm

Unresponsive?
Not breathing or
only occasional gasps

Call
resuscitation team

CPR 30:2
Attach defibrillator/monitor
Minimise interruptions

Assess
rhythm

Shockable
(VF/Pulseless VT)

Non-Shockable
(PEA/Asystole)

1 Shock

Return of
spontaneous
circulation

Immediately resume
CPR for 2 min
Minimise interruptions

**Immediate post cardiac
arrest treatment**
• Use ABCDE approach
• Controlled oxygenation and
  ventilation
• 12-lead ECG
• Treat precipitating cause
• Temperature control/
  therapeutic hypothermia

Immediately resume
CPR for 2 min
Minimise interruptions

During CPR
• Ensure high-quality CPR: rate, depth, recoil
• Plan actions before interrupting CPR
• Give oxygen
• Consider advanced airway and capnography
• Continuous chest compressions when
  advanced airway in place
• Vascular access (intravenous, intraosseous)
• Give adrenaline every 3–5 min
• Correct reversible causes

Reversible Causes
• Hypoxia
• Hypovolaemia
• Hypo-/hyperkalaemia/metabolic
• Hypothermia

• Thrombosis – coronary or pulmonary
• Tamponade – cardiac
• Toxins
• Tension pneumothorax

FIGURE 1.3 Cardiac arrest. Reproduced with the kind permission of the
Resuscitation Council (UK).

Case 14

The ECG demonstrates evidence of low voltage complexes. In view of the history and examination findings, the most likely diagnosis is cardiac tamponade. The patient should be stabilised using the 'ABC' approach and undergo an urgent pericardiocentesis.

Case 15

The chest X-ray demonstrates cardiomegaly with ill-defined pulmonary vasculature in keeping with mild pulmonary oedema.

Based on the presentation and chest X-ray the most likely diagnosis is heart failure.

According to NICE, patients should undergo B type natriuretic peptide (BNP) measurement as well as an ECHO. A BNP level less than 100 pg/mL is deemed normal.

NICE advises the use of ACE inhibitors and beta blockers as first-line treatment. An aldosterone antagonist is often used in cases of moderate to severe heart failure (New York Heart Association (NYHA) III–IV). In individuals of African or Caribbean origin the use of hydralazine in combination with nitrates may prove worthwhile in NYHA III–IV. In case of persistent symptoms patients should be offered cardiac resynchronisation therapy or digoxin.

2 Endocrinology

Case 1

The glucose results confirm a diagnosis of diabetes. According to the WHO the following criteria are used:

Diabetes	
Fasting plasma glucose	≥7.0 mmol/L or
2-hour plasma glucose	≥11.1 mmol/L
Impaired glucose tolerance (IGT)	
Fasting plasma glucose	<7.0 mmol/L and
2-hour plasma glucose	≥7.8 and <11.1 mmol/L
Impaired fasting glucose (IFG)	
Fasting plasma glucose	6.1–6.9 mmol/L and
2-hour plasma glucose	<7.8 mmol/L

Two-hour plasma glucose is measured after ingestion of 75 g oral glucose. In view of the negative anti-GAD antibodies, the most likely diagnosis is Type II diabetes. According to NICE the management of Type II diabetes commonly starts with metformin following an HbA1c of 6.5% after life-style interventions. Sulphonylureas are commenced instead if individuals are not overweight and if metformin is not tolerated or is contraindicated. Metformin and sulphonylureas may be used in combination in cases where the HBA1c remains higher than 6.5% despite the use of metformin initially. If the HBA1c following such intervention remains above 7.5%, then insulin is added. If there is risk of hypoglycaemia with the use of sulphonylureas, then one could consider the use of a DPP-4 inhibitor or thiazolidinedione. If there are issues with regard to the use of insulin in view of obesity, for example, then one can choose to use sitagliptin as an alternative. In addition to anti-diabetic medication, clinicians should focus on the control of blood lipids and optimum blood pressure control.

Points to note
- Metformin can result in GI side effects. Metformin should be stopped if the serum creatinine > 150 mcmol/L.
- Sulphonylureas are associated with renal dysfunction and hypoglycaemia.
- Thiazolidinediones should be avoided in those with heart failure or at risk of fracture.

Case 2

The results demonstrate a phenomenon known as sick euthyroid syndrome. Essentially this is a presentation whereby individuals present with abnormal thyroid function occurring on a background of non-thyroidal illness. One typically observes a reduction in TSH, T4 and T3. The condition can occur during systemic illness and can typically be seen in intensive-care patients. There are no current guidelines on the management of sick euthyroid syndrome and it is still unclear as to whether the use of thyroid replacement is of much use.

Case 3

In view of the normal T4 and elevated TSH, the diagnosis in this case is subclinical hypothyroidism. It is generally felt that individuals with a TSH greater than 10 mU/L should be treated with thyroxine, due to the risk of eventually developing overt hypothyroidism.

Case 4

In view of the low serum calcium, elevated parathyroid hormone and impaired renal function the most likely diagnosis is secondary hyperparathyroidism. In chronic renal failure, there is overproduction of parathyroid hormone in view of excess phosphate production, low serum calcium and impaired vitamin D production. The management of secondary hyperparathyroidism involves vitamin D and calcium replacement and the use of phosphate binders. Surgical intervention is employed in cases of secondary hyperparathyroidism refractory to medical intervention.

Case 5

In view of the low calcium and low parathyroid hormone the most likely diagnosis is primary hypoparathyroidism. The seizure activity is secondary to the low calcium. The condition often occurs following parathyroidectomy and is also autoimmune related. Management relies on replacement of calcium and vitamin D.

Case 6

In view of the positive dexamethasone and late night salivary cortisol test, the most likely diagnosis is Cushing's syndrome. The Endocrine Society states that a diagnosis of Cushing's syndrome occurs when there is an abnormal urinary free cortisol, serum cortisol greater than 1.8 mcg/dL after 1 mg dexamethasone and late night salivary cortisol greater than 145 ng/dL.

Case 7

In view of the history and cortisol findings post synacthen, the most likely diagnosis is Addison's disease. The lack of serum cortisol also helps to explain the low sodium and high potassium. Addison's disease is excluded if the serum cortisol rises above 550 nmol/L (20 mcg/dL) 30 minutes post synacthen.

Case 8

The urine osmolality after ADH has not changed, implying nephrogenic diabetes insipidus. In cranial diabetes insipidus, the urine osmolality increases to more than 750 mosmol/kg after ADH. In primary polydipsia the urine osmolality after water deprivation is typically above 750 mosmol/kg.

Case 9

In view of the history and blood investigations, the most likely diagnosis is diabetic ketoacidosis (DKA). According to the Joint British Diabetes Societies, the diagnostic criteria for a DKA include:
- a capillary blood glucose above 11 mmol/L
- capillary ketones above 3 mmol/L or urine ketones ++ or more
- venous pH less than 7.3 and/or bicarbonate less than 15 mmol/L.

Patients should be commenced on IV sodium chloride and an insulin infusion, typically 50 units of human soluble insulin in 50 mL of 0.9% sodium chloride at a rate of 0.1 units/kg/hr. Intravenous fluid replacement is blood pressure dependent. Individuals with a systolic below 90 mmHg should be given 500 mL of 0.9% sodium chloride over 10–15 minutes. If systolic BP is above 90, then 1 L of sodium chloride should be given over the first 60 minutes. Potassium replacement is level dependent:
- potassium > 5.5 mmol – nil
- potassium > 3.5–5.5 mmol/L – 40 mmol/L
- potassium < 3.5 mmol – requires HDU intervention.

Over the next 60 minutes to 6 hours, fluid should be replaced as follows:
- 0.9% sodium chloride 1 L with potassium chloride over next 2 hours
- 0.9% sodium chloride 1 L with potassium chloride over next 2 hours
- 0.9% sodium chloride 1 L with potassium chloride over next 4 hours
- add 10% glucose 125 mL/hr if blood glucose falls below 14 mmol/L.

From 6 to 12 hours, fluid should be adjusted at a reduced rate:
- 0.9% sodium chloride 1 L with potassium chloride over 4 hours
- 0.9% sodium chloride 1 L with potassium chloride over 6 hours
- add 10% glucose 125 mL/hr if blood glucose falls below 14 mmol/L.

Throughout patient management, appropriate monitoring of blood glucose, ketones, pH, bicarbonate and potassium should occur. A DKA is regarded as resolved when ketones are <0.3 mmol/L and venous pH is >7.3.

Case 10

In view of the history and blood investigations, the most likely diagnosis is hyperosmolar hyperglycaemic state (HHS). According to the Joint British Diabetes Societies, the characteristic features of HHS are:
- hypovolaemia
- marked hyperglycaemia (30 mmol/L or more) without significant hyperketonaemia (<3 mmol/L) or acidosis (pH > 7.3, bicarbonate > 15 mmol/L)
- osmolality usually 320 mosmol/kg or more.

The treatment of HHS relies upon the following parameters:
- using intravenous (IV) 0.9% sodium chloride solution as the principle fluid to restore circulating volume and reverse dehydration
- a fall in blood glucose, which should be no more than 5 mmol/L/hr. Low dose IV insulin (0.05 units/kg/hr) should only be commenced once the blood glucose is no longer falling with IV fluids alone OR immediately if there is significant ketonaemia
- IV fluid replacement to achieve a positive balance of 3–6 L by 12 hours and the remaining replacement of estimated fluid losses within the next 12 hours, though complete normalisation of biochemistry may take up to 72 hours
- the use of prophylactic anticoagulation in most patients.

3 Gastroenterology

Case 1

The CT demonstrates evidence of an enlarged cirrhotic liver with a large hepatocellular carcinoma occupying a substantial portion of the right lobe of the liver in addition to portal vein thrombosis and adjacent lymphadenopathy.

Liver function tests including serum alpha-fetoprotein (AFP) are essential blood investigations. AFP tends to be raised in up to 75% of cases. A chest X-ray may be useful to exclude pulmonary metastases. Biopsy under CT or ultrasound guidance is rarely required.

According to the British Society of Gastroenterology (BSG), the mainstay form of treatment is surgery for patients with a single small liver cancer less than 5 cm or those with up to three liver lesions less than 3 cm. Ethanol injection has been shown to produce necrosis of peripheral lesions less than 3 cm in diameter. Radiofrequency ablation is a useful alternative.

Case 2

The X-ray demonstrates evidence of thickening of the descending and sigmoid colon in keeping with active colitis. In view of the fact that the patient complained of bloody stools, the most likely diagnosis is ulcerative colitis, although an endoscopy would be required to confirm this histologically.

Investigations of choice include a full blood count, urea and electrolytes, liver function tests, serum albumin, glucose and CRP, as well as haematinics. Stools should be sent for *Clostridium difficile* (*C. difficile*) and microscopy and culture. Within 72 hours, patients should undergo a flexible sigmoidoscopy and biopsy, and an abdominal X-ray should be repeated if there is any change in the patient's condition.

Taking into consideration the history, examination and investigation findings, this patient would be classified as suffering from acute **severe** ulcerative colitis. The Truelove and Witts' criteria defines colitis as follows:

Features	Mild	Moderate	Severe
Motions/day	<4	4–6	>6
Temperature (°C)	Apyrexial	37.1–37.8	>37.8
Pulse rate (beats per minute)	<70	70–90	>90
Haemoglobin (g/dL)	>11	10.5–11	<10.5
ESR (mm/hr)	<20	20–30	>30

In accordance with the BSG, management relies on the use of IV fluids and electrolyte replacement with blood transfusion to maintain an Hb >10 g/dL. Subcutaneous heparin helps to reduce the risk of thromboembolism. Intravenous corticosteroids in the form of hydrocortisone 100 mg four times a day are the mainstay form of treatment. If after commencing steroid therapy there is no improvement after day three, a colectomy or treatment with intravenous ciclosporin or infliximab should be considered. Surgery is also a priority in cases of toxic megacolon.

Case 3

The CT demonstrates evidence of free fluid, gallstones and inflammatory changes in the pancreas in keeping with acute pancreatitis.

In addition to an abdominal CT scan, serum amylase and lipase are useful investigations.

Patients with acute pancreatitis should be assessed according to severity. Features that may predict a severe attack within 48 hours of admission to hospital include the patient's clinical state, a Glasgow score of 3 or more, a CRP of more than 150 mg/L, persisting organ failure for 48 hours, and the presence of progressive organ failure.

The Glasgow score comprises the following parameters:

$PO_2 < 7.9$ kPa
Age > 55 years
White cell count $> 15 \times 10^9$/L
Calcium < 2 mmol/L
Urea > 16 mmol/L
LDH > 600 U/L
Albumin < 32 g/L
Serum glucose > 10 mmol/L

According to the BSG, the use of antibiotics in acute pancreatitis is not concrete. If antibiotics are used, they should be continued for a 14-day period. Feeding via the enteral route is also important. In cases of pancreatitis secondary to gallstones, patients should undergo therapeutic ERCP. In cases of infected necrosis, patients will require debridement.

Case 4

There is marked distension of the large bowel in keeping with large bowel obstruction.

A full blood count and renal function are important blood investigations. In addition to an abdominal X-ray, a CT scan may be helpful but is not always indicated.

Patients with large bowel obstruction require fluid resuscitation, NG tube insertion for decompression purposes as well as surgical intervention.

Below is an abdominal X-ray of a patient with small bowel obstruction for comparison.

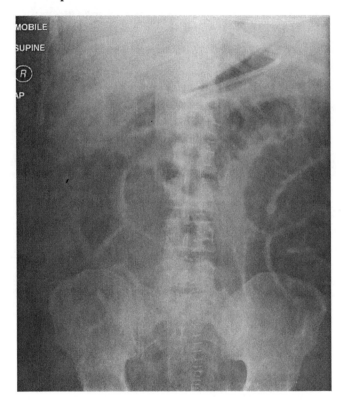

Case 5

Based on the history and histology report, the diagnosis in this case is a gastric ulcer secondary to *Helicobacter pylori* (*H. pylori*).

According to NICE, patients with gastric ulcers should stop any drug that could worsen symptoms such as NSAIDs, steroids, theophyllines, bisphosphonates, calcium channel blockers and nitrates. Lifestyle advice should also be offered in terms of weight loss and smoking cessation. If *H. pylori* is present, patients should be treated with a PPI, amoxicillin and clarithromycin, or a PPI with metronidazole and clarithromycin for 7 days as eradication therapy. PPIs should generally be continued for up to 2 months. After treatment patients should undergo a repeat endoscopy.

Patients with a gastric ulcer, who are negative for *H. pylori*, should simply be treated with a PPI for up to 2 months.

Case 6

The histology report indicates the presence of *C. difficile*, most likely due to the antibiotics commenced for treatment of the patient's pneumonia. Stool cultures in the first instance are essential as opposed to an endoscopy.

In accordance with the European Society of Clinical Microbiology and Infectious Diseases (ESCMID), patients with mild *C. difficile* infection, namely a stool frequency of less than four times daily, secondary to antibiotics and with no signs of severe colitis can be treated by simply stopping the antibiotic. Features of severe colitis include:

- fever >38.5 °C
- rigors
- haemodynamic instability
- peritonism
- signs of ileus
- a leucocyte count of $>15 \times 10^9/L$
- an increase in creatinine >50% above the baseline
- the existence of pseudomembranous colitis following colonoscopy or sigmoidoscopy.

In all other cases antibiotic therapy should be started comprising of metronidazole in non-severe cases or vancomycin in severe cases. Metronidazole can be given intravenously when oral therapy is not possible. An alternative to vancomycin is teicoplanin.

Surgical intervention for *C. difficile* should be performed in cases of colonic perforation, deterioration in clinical state as well as toxic megacolon and ileus.

Case 7

The blood investigations demonstrate a fall in Hb, a rise in the platelet count and inflammatory markers. There is also a rise in serum urea. Taking into consideration the history, the patient is suffering from an upper GI bleed.

In accordance with NICE, patients presenting with an upper GI bleed should undergo Blatchford scoring at first assessment and the Rockall score post endoscopy.

Blatchford scoring criteria

Admission risk marker	Score component value
Blood urea (mmol/L)	
≥6.5 <8.0	2
≥8.0 <10.0	3
≥10.0 <25·0	4
≥25	6
Haemoglobin (g/dL) for men	
≥12.0 <13.0	1
≥10.0 <12.0	3
<10.0	6
Haemoglobin (g/dL) for women	
≥10.0 <12.0	1
<10.0	6
Systolic blood pressure (mmHg)	
100–109	1
90–99	2
<90	3
Other markers	
Pulse ≥100 (per min)	1
Presentation with melaena	1
Presentation with syncope	2
Hepatic disease	2
Cardiac failure	2

A score of 6 or more is associated with a 50% risk of requiring an intervention such as a transfusion, endoscopy or surgery.

The Rockall score criteria

Variable	0	1	2	3	
Age	<60	60–79	>80		
Shock	No shock	Tachycardia, pulse > 100 beats per minute	Hypotension, SBP < 100 mmHg		Initial Score
Comorbidity	No major comorbidity		Cardiac failure, IHD, any major comorbidity	Renal failure, liver failure, disseminated malignancy	
Diagnosis	Mallory–Weiss tear, no lesion identified and no stigmata of recent haemorrhage	All other diagnoses	Malignancy of upper GI tract		Additional criteria for full score
Major stigmata of recent haemorrhage	None, or dark spot only		Blood in upper GI tract, adherent clot, visible or spurting vessel		

In accordance with the fall in Hb, patients should be transfused accordingly. NICE recommends that platelets should be given to those with a platelet count of less than 50×10^9/L and who are actively bleeding. Fresh frozen plasma (FFP) should be given to those with a fibrinogen of less than 1 g/L or a PT or APTT greater than 1.5 times normal. Prothrombin complex should be offered to patients taking warfarin and who are actively bleeding.

For non-variceal bleeds, patients should be treated with mechanical clips, thermal coagulation, or fibrin with or without adrenaline. Proton pump inhibitors should then be commenced after treatment. For variceal bleeds, band ligation should be used initially in cases of oesophageal varices. Transjugular intrahepatic portosystemic shunt (TIPS) is recommended in cases where bleeding is not controlled following banding.

Gastric varices are best treated with N–butyl-2-cyanoacrylate.

Case 8

The blood results demonstrate a rise in the white cell count and thrombocytopenia with deranged renal and liver function as well as hypoglycaemia. Together with confusion, one can conclude the existence of acute liver failure. The confusion would be evident of encephalopathy.

Further blood investigations of use include serum magnesium, phosphate and ammonia. An arterial blood gas will provide information regarding lactate level and the presence of acidosis. Additional tests include blood cultures, a paracetamol level, hepatitis screen, toxicology screen, autoimmune screen and ceruloplasmin level. A liver ultrasound and/or CT are worthwhile imaging techniques. And a liver biopsy may help to ascertain underlying pathology. However, such a procedure is not undertaken in the coagulopathy setting.

It is advised that the management of patients with acute liver failure occurs in the ITU setting. A CT brain helps to exclude other causes of altered mental status and patients must refrain from being sedated. Antibiotics should be used in cases of infection as well as lactulose. In cases of hyponatremia, patients may benefit from hypertonic saline. Vitamin K is used in cases of coagulopathy with FFP and platelets in case of active bleeding. In cases of renal failure, haemodialysis may be employed and patients should be given appropriate nutritional support.

Case 9

The blood results demonstrate evidence of hepatitis in addition to a positive IgG, ANA and anti-smooth muscle antibodies (ASMA). In view of the history and examination findings the most likely diagnosis is autoimmune hepatitis.

According to the BSG, patients should undergo liver function tests and serum immunoglobulins. Serum gamma globulin and IgG are elevated in most cases. In cases of type I autoimmune hepatitis, there may be a positive ANA and ASMAs. In type II, there may be a positive anti-LKM-1 antibody and anti-LC-1 antibody. A liver biopsy is essential in terms of making a diagnosis, which will show evidence of interface hepatitis with or without bridging necrosis.

The BSG recommends the use of prednisolone in addition to azathioprine. Patients intolerant of prednisolone are best managed with budesonide. In view of the risk of osteoporosis whilst on steroids, patients require calcium and vitamin D supplementation. Referral for a liver transplant is advised for those patients who respond slowly to treatment and in those who present with fulminant hepatic failure.

Case 10

Based on the histology report, the most likely diagnosis is Crohn's disease. In accordance with the BSG, patients with severe Crohn's disease should be treated with intravenous steroids. Those with moderately active Crohn's should be commenced on prednisolone up to 40 mg daily, which is then tapered depending on response. Patients who are refractory to steroids should be commenced on anti-TNF-alpha therapy. Other agents capable of inducing remission are azathioprine, 6-MP and methotrexate.

Case 11

Based on the history and investigations shown, the most likely diagnosis is coeliac disease. There is evidence of anaemia, electrolyte deficiencies and a low albumin in addition to a prolonged prothrombin time, which is likely due to malabsorption of vitamin K. The most sensitive and specific test is tissue transglutaminase IgA antibody. An endoscopy is also key, with biopsy findings demonstrating evidence of crypt hyperplasia, villous atrophy and an increase in intraepithelial lymphocytes.

Case 12

The results demonstrate acute hepatitis B infection. In general, the presence of the HBsAg, in addition to the HBeAg, anti-HBc, IgM anti-HBc, HBV DNA and abnormal ALT implies acute pathology.

Acute hepatitis B is typically managed with pain relief and anti-emetics. Anti-virals are not required in acute cases unless progression to fulminant hepatitis has occurred. Hepatitis B is a notifiable disease and hence the Health Protection Unit must be informed.

With regard to chronic hepatitis B infection, the main drug treatments of choice are pegylated interferon, nucleoside analogues (lamivudine, telbivudine, entecavir) and nucleotide analogues (adefovir and tenofovir).

4 Neurology

Case 1

The CT demonstrates a large haemorrhage in the right parieto-occipital region.

In view of the history and CT findings the most likely diagnosis is a stroke. NICE advocates the following with regard to management:

- Brain imaging should occur immediately if any of the following applies:
  - indications for thrombolysis or early anticoagulation treatment
  - on anticoagulant treatment
  - a known bleeding tendency
  - a depressed level of consciousness (Glasgow Coma Score [GCS] <13)
  - unexplained progressive or fluctuating symptoms
  - papilloedema, neck stiffness or fever
  - severe headache at onset of stroke symptoms.
- In cases of an ischaemic stroke, thrombolysis with alteplase is preferred within the first 3 hours of symptom onset. If this time window has elapsed, then aspirin 300 mg should be given. In cases of a haemorrhagic stroke, aspirin should not be used.
- Nutrition should be optimised usually with an NG tube in cases of dysphagia and risk of aspiration. Blood glucose should be maintained between 4 and 11 mmol/L and blood pressure controlled in case of the following:
  - hypertensive encephalopathy
  - hypertensive nephropathy
  - hypertensive cardiac failure/myocardial infarction
  - aortic dissection
  - pre-eclampsia/eclampsia
  - intracerebral haemorrhage with a systolic blood pressure of >200 mmHg.
- In this case the patient has had a haemorrhagic stroke and hence should be referred to neurosurgical specialists as appropriate.

Case 2

In view of the CSF findings and history, the most likely diagnosis is multiple sclerosis (MS) (note the presence of the oligoclonal bands).

NICE advocates the use of methylprednisolone during the acute phase of multiple sclerosis. For those with relapsing-remitting multiple sclerosis, the Association of British Neurologists (ABN) advises the use of interferon beta for those who:

* can walk 100 metres or more without assistance
* have had at least two clinically significant relapses in the past 2 years
* are aged 18 years or older
* do not have contraindications.

Glatiramer acetate should be used for relapsing-remitting MS for those who:

* can walk 100 metres or more without assistance
* have had at least two clinically significant relapses in the past 2 years
* are aged 18 years or older
* do not have contraindications.

In cases of secondary progressive MS, patients should be treated with interferon beta if they:

* can walk 10 metres or more with or without assistance
* have had at least two disabling relapses in the past 2 years
* have had minimal increase in disability due to gradual progression over the past 2 years
* are aged over 18 years
* do not have contraindications.

Case 3

The schematic demonstrates a decline in action potential amplitude over time with some minimal improvement as time progresses. This is in keeping with myasthenia gravis.

The management of such a condition relies on the use of acetylcholinesterase inhibitors such as pyridostigmine, steroids and azathioprine. The use of IvIg, plasmapheresis and thymectomy also play a significant role.

Case 4

In view of the predominance of polymorphs, low glucose and elevated opening pressure, the most likely diagnosis is bacterial meningitis. The treatment of choice is ceftriaxone IV.

Learning Point

It is important to realise that such a condition can alter a patient's state significantly, particularly from a sepsis perspective. If the patient presents as significantly septic, the following should be noted:

- Resuscitation should be started in patients who are hypotensive and with a lactate of >4 mmol/L, targeted to achieve a CVP of 8–12 mmHg, a MAP >65 mmHg, urine output >0.5 mL/kg/hr and central venous saturations >70%. If venous saturations are not achieved transfuse further fluid, packed red blood cells to achieve a haematocrit >30% and start a dobutamine infusion.
- Blood cultures are essential in a septic patient and should be obtained ideally before starting antibiotics.
- Fluid resuscitation is ideally with crystalloids or colloids, and vasopressors can be used to achieve the appropriate MAP with norepinephrine and dopamine. In cases of myocardial dysfunction, patients should be started on dobutamine.
- Intravenous hydrocortisone is often started on patients when hypotension responds poorly to fluid and vasopressors.

Case 5

In view of the history, raised lymphocyte count, elevated protein and normal glucose the most likely diagnosis is viral encephalitis. Acyclovir is the treatment of choice.

5 Overdose

Case 1

The arterial blood gas initially demonstrates a respiratory alkalosis and later a metabolic acidosis. In view of the history the most likely diagnosis is salicylate poisoning.

In cases of mild poisoning (salicylate level of 300–600 mg/L), oral or intravenous fluids are the treatment of choice. For moderate poisoning (salicylate level of 600–800 mg/L), urinary alkalinisation with sodium bicarbonate is preferred. In cases of severe poisoning (level > 800 mg/L), haemodialysis is the treatment of choice.

Case 2

In view of the history and blood results, the most likely diagnosis is a paracetamol overdose. The MHRA advocate the use of acetylcysteine in the following circumstances:

- Paracetamol overdose irrespective of the plasma paracetamol level in circumstances where the overdose is staggered or there is doubt over the time of paracetamol ingestion; or

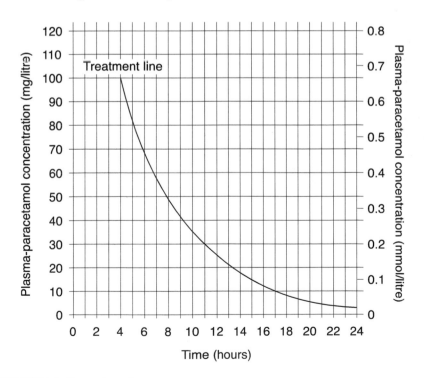

FIGURE 5.1 Paracetamol nomogram

- Paracetamol overdose with a timed plasma paracetamol concentration on or above a single treatment line joining points of 100 mg/L at 4 hours and 15 mg/L at 15 hours of the nomogram, regardless of risk factors of hepatotoxicity.
- An increase in the duration of administration of the first dose of intravenous acetylcysteine from 15 minutes to 1 hour.

The King's College criteria help to determine which patients who suffer from paracetamol-induced liver failure are at high risk from mortality and hence would benefit from a liver transplant:
- pH < 7.30
- and all three of:
  - INR > 6.5
  - serum creatinine > 300 mcmol/L
  - the presence of grade 3 or 4 encephalopathy.

6 Renal

Case 1

There is evidence of a right retroperitoneal haematoma. The major complication of a renal biopsy is bleeding post procedure. Additional complications include pain and arteriovenous fistula formation.

Case 2

The blood results demonstrate evidence of worsening renal function in keeping with acute kidney injury. The Renal Association (RA) defines acute kidney injury (AKI) when one of the following criteria are met:

- serum creatinine rises by ≥26 mcmol/L within 48 hours; or
- serum creatinine rises ≥1.5 fold from the reference value, which is known or presumed to have occurred within 1 week; or
- urine output is <0.5 mL/kg/hr for >6 consecutive hours.

The reference serum creatinine should be the lowest creatinine value recorded within 3 months of the event.

In accordance with the RA, the following investigations are useful: urea and electrolytes, full blood count, urinalysis (± microscopy), urine culture (if infection is suspected), blood cultures (if infection is suspected), renal immunology and urinary electrolytes and osmolality. In addition, patients should have an ECG, chest X-ray, abdominal X-ray, a renal tract ultrasound within 24 hours of presentation and be considered for a renal biopsy.

Fluids should be instigated following assessment of patient's volume status. Nephrotoxic medications should be stopped and patient's usual medications should be dosed accordingly. Patients with AKI should receive 25–35 kcal/kg/day and up to a maximum of 1.7 g amino acids/kg/day if hypercatabolic and receiving continuous renal replacement therapy. From the case described, there is evidence of hyperkalaemia, which should be treated with calcium gluconate, which is cardioprotective, insulin/dextrose, salbutamol nebulisers and calcium resonium.

The decision to commence renal replacement therapy relies upon meeting the following parameters:

Biochemical indications
- Refractory hyperkalaemia > 6.5 mmol/L.
- Serum urea > 27 mmol/L.
- Refractory metabolic acidosis pH < 7.15.
- Refractory electrolyte abnormalities:

  ‣ hyponatraemia, hypernatraemia or hypercalcaemia.
  ‣ tumour lysis syndrome with hyperuricaemia and hyperphosphataemia.
  ‣ urea cycle defects, and organic acidurias resulting in hyperammonaemia, methylmalonic acidaemia.

Clinical indications
- Urine output < 0.3 mL/kg for 24 hours or absolute anuria for 12 hours.
- AKI with multiple organ failure.
- Refractory volume overload.
- End organ involvement: pericarditis, encephalopathy, neuropathy, myopathy, uraemic bleeding.
- Creation of intravascular space for plasma and other blood product infusions and nutrition.
- Severe poisoning or drug overdose.
- Severe hypothermia or hyperthermia.

Case 3
From the history and investigations, the most likely diagnosis is nephrotic syndrome. Patients should have a urine microscopy and culture. Urine should be sent for protein–creatinine ratio (PCR) with >300 mg/mmol being diagnostic of nephrotic syndrome. Other useful tests include an autoimmune screen, chest X-ray, renal ultrasound, Doppler ultrasound to exclude thrombosis and renal biopsy.

The management of nephrotic syndrome relies on the use of sodium restriction, diuretics and limited fluid intake. Diuretics of choice include both loop and thiazide diuretics. ACE inhibitors help to reduce the degree of proteinuria.

Case 4

The history and blood investigations are in keeping with chronic kidney disease (CKD). CKD can be classified as follows:

Stage	eGFR (mL/min/1.73 m²)	Description
1	>90	Normal or increased GFR, with other evidence of kidney damage
2	60–89	Slight decrease in GFR, with other evidence of kidney damage
3A	45–59	Moderate decrease in GFR, with or without other evidence of kidney damage
3B	30–44	Moderate decrease in GFR, with or without other evidence of kidney damage
4	15–29	Severe decrease in GFR, with or without other evidence of kidney damage
5	<15	Established renal failure

NICE advises the use of a renal ultrasound in patients with CKD who:
- have progressive CKD
- have visible or persistent invisible haematuria
- have symptoms of urinary tract obstruction
- have a family history of polycystic kidney disease and are aged over 20
- have stage 4 or 5 CKD
- are considered by a nephrologist to require a renal biopsy.

Blood pressure should be kept below 140/90 mmHg and in diabetics below 130/80 mmHg. Individuals should be offered bisphosphonates for the prevention and treatment of osteoporosis and vitamin D supplementation as needed.

Diabetic patients with an albumin–creatinine ratio (ACR) >2.5 mg/mmol (men) or 3.5 mg/mmol (women) with or without hypertension should be treated with ACE inhibitors. In non-diabetics, if the ACR is >70 mg/mmol with or without hypertension, offer ACE inhibitors.

Case 5

In view of the history and blood investigations, this boy is suffering from haemolytic uraemic syndrome (HUS) secondary to *E. coli* 0157. The triad of HUS comprises microangiopathic haemolytic anaemia, thrombocytopenia and acute renal failure. The blood film shows evidence of helmet-shaped cells called schistocytes. The treatment of choice is fluid resuscitation and plasma exchange.

Case 6

In view of the results obtained and the history, the most likely diagnosis is syndrome of inappropriate ADH (SIADH). This is due to the presence of a high urinary concentration and urine osmolality in addition to hyponatraemia and a low plasma osmolality. Treatment of choice includes fluid restriction, the use of loop diuretics and vasopressin receptor antagonists. Demeclocycline is not commonly used.

Case 7

The ECG demonstrates evidence of a widened QRS and peaked T waves in keeping with hyperkalaemia. This is likely to be due to acute renal failure in view of the patient's reduced urinary frequency most likely secondary to obstruction. The treatment of hyperkalaemia involves calcium gluconate (cardioprotective), insulin/dextrose, salbutamol nebulisers and calcium resonium. The treatment of acute renal failure in general is discussed in a previous case.

Case 8

This patient has an elevated total cholesterol and LDL cholesterol. According to the Simon Broome criteria, this is in keeping with familial hypercholesterolaemia (FH).

1   Total cholesterol >7.5 mmol/L or low-density lipoprotein (LDL) cholesterol >4.9 mmol/L in adults
2   Tendon xanthomas are present in the patient, first-degree relative or second-degree relative
3   DNA-based evidence of a mutation in the LDL receptor, Apo B-100 or PCSK9
4   Family history of premature myocardial infarction (<50 years in second-degree relative or <60 years in first-degree relative
5   Family history of elevated total cholesterol (>7.5 mmol/L in first- or second-degree relative)

The management of familial hypercholesterolaemia relies on the use of stains or ezetimibe if statins are not tolerated. Patients should also stop smoking, maintain a healthy diet, increase physical activity and limit their alcohol intake.

Case 9

The ECG demonstrates evidence of a prolonged QT interval. This is likely to be due to hypocalcaemia, which is common in acute pancreatitis. The management of hypocalcaemia relies upon oral replacement or intravenous calcium gluconate in severe cases. The management of acute pancreatitis is discussed in a previous case.

7 Haematology

Case 1

The results demonstrate evidence of a microcytic hypochromic anaemia with a low ferritin in keeping with iron deficiency anaemia. The BSG recognises iron deficiency anaemia by the presence of a low serum ferritin, red cell microcytosis or hypochromia in the absence of chronic disease or haemoglobinopathies. The BSG advises screening for coeliac disease in addition to upper and lower GI investigations for female patients who are post-menopausal, aged over 50 and have a strong family history of colorectal cancer and all male patients where iron deficiency has been confirmed.

The treatment of iron deficiency anaemia involves iron supplementation either orally (iron sulphate 200 mg) or parenterally in cases where oral preparations are not tolerated. Blood transfusions are offered in cases of cardiovascular instability due to the degree of anaemia.

Case 2

The patient has evidence of microcytic anaemia with a raised ferritin in keeping with sideroblastic anaemia. Basophilic stippling is commonly seen in cases of lead poisoning, which is a cause of sideroblastic anaemia. Management relies on treatment of the underlying cause in addition to the use of folic acid, pyridoxine and blood transfusions.

Case 3

The history and investigations demonstrate evidence of hypereosinophilic syndrome associated with an eosinophil count greater than $1.5 \times 10^9/L$. Management relies on the use of steroids as the first line for those without the FIP1L1-PDGFRA genotype. Those with this genotype benefit from imatinib.

Case 4

Evidence of a macrocytic anaemia in addition to normal urinary measurements of radiolabelled B_{12} following intrinsic factor implies pernicious anaemia. In this case without intrinsic factor, B_{12} is unable to be absorbed and excreted in the urine. However, following intrinsic factor this malabsorption is normalised. This is the basis of the Schilling's test. Management of pernicious anaemia relies on treatment of the underlying cause and the use of vitamin B_{12} replacement.

Case 5

The results demonstrate a macrocytic anaemia with increased bilirubin and LDH in keeping with haemolytic anaemia. The increased MCV is due to increased red cell production (reticulocytosis). The treatment of haemolytic anaemia depends on the underlying cause and relies on the replacement of folic acid as well as steroids and IvIg in autoimmune cases.

Case 6

The history and blood results are in keeping with a sickle cell crisis, in view of the elevated bilirubin, reticulocyte count and target cells.

Additional investigations would include:
- chest radiograph (febrile, breathless, tachypnoea, chest pain, chest signs, reduced oxygen saturations)
- arterial blood gases (oxygen saturations <95%, unexplained drowsiness)
- blood and urine cultures (febrile, rigors, hypotensive)
- ultrasound abdomen (abnormal LFTs, abdominal pain, splenomegaly)
- parvovirus B19 serology (reticulocytopenia)
- computerised tomography / magnetic resonance imaging (MRI) scans of brain (if seizure, transient ischaemic attack, stroke, severe headache).

The British Committee for Standards in Haematology (BCSH) advise that analgesia should be given within 30 minutes of entering the hospital and effective analgesia achieved by 60 minutes. Pain, respiratory rate and sedation should be assessed every 20 minutes until pain is controlled.

Pain management is governed by the WHO analgesic ladder:

Step 1: mild pain
- Non-opioid ± adjuvant.

Step 2: moderate pain
- Weak opioid (or low dose of strong opioid) ± non-opioid ± adjuvant.

Step 3: severe pain
- Strong opioid ± non-opioid ± adjuvant.

The management of acute pain in opioid-naïve adults is depicted below:
1 Rapid clinical assessment.
2 If pain severe and oral analgesia not effective, give strong opioids:
   ‣ morphine 0.1 mg/kg IV/SC repeated every 20 minutes until pain controlled
   ‣ then 0.05–0.1 mg/kg every 2–4 hours IV/SC/PO – consider PCA

Or diamorphine 0.1 mg/kg IV/SC repeated every 20 minutes until pain controlled
  ▶ then 0.05–0.1 mg/kg every 2–4 h IV/SC – consider PCA.
3 Give adjuvant non-opioid analgesia: paracetamol, ibuprofen, diclofenac, ketorolac.
4 Prescribe laxatives routinely and other adjuvants as necessary:
  ▶ laxatives: lactulose 10 mL/bd, senna 2–4 tablets od, docusate 100 mg bd
  ▶ antipruritics: hydroxyzine 25 mg bd
  ▶ antiemetics: prochlorperazine 5–10 mg tds, cyclizine 50 mg tds
  ▶ anxiolytic: haloperidol 1–3 mg PO/IM bd.
5 Monitor pain, sedation, vital signs, respiratory rate and oxygen saturations every 30 minutes until pain controlled and stable, and then every 2 hours.
6 Give rescue doses of analgesia every 30 minutes for breakthrough pains: 50% of maintenance dose.
7 If respiratory rate less than 10/min, omit maintenance analgesia. If severe respiratory depression/sedation, give 100 mcg naloxone IV, repeating every 2 minutes as necessary.
8 Consider reducing analgesia after 2–3 days and replacing injections with equivalent dose of oral opiate.
9 Discharge patient when pain controlled and improving without analgesia or on acceptable doses of oral analgesia.
10 Arrange any necessary home care and an outpatient follow-up appointment.

Non-pharmacological management relies upon fluid replacement. Intravenous fluids should not be used routinely, but should be given if the patient is unable to drink, is vomiting or has diarrhoea. Nasogastric fluids should be considered as an alternative to intravenous fluids.

Oxygen should not be used routinely, but is appropriate if the oxygen saturation is less than 95%.

Broad-spectrum antibiotics should be used if the patient is febrile (temperature > 38 °C), systemically unwell, or has chest symptoms.

Blood transfusions should not be used as a treatment for pain, but are important for symptomatic anaemia. Blood for transfusion should be leucodepleted and matched for Rh and Kell antigens.

Incentive spirometry should be used for patients with chest or back pain.

Patients should be monitored every 2 hours for pain control (using a pain chart), sedation, respiratory rate and oxygen saturation, and every 4 hours for temperature and pulse.

Case 7

In view of the isolated thrombocytopenia, the most likely diagnosis is idiopathic thrombocytopenic purpura (ITP), which is common following a viral illness. The mainstay form of treatment is steroids and as a second-line IvIg. Research has also shown promising results with rituximab. From a surgical perspective, splenectomy is associated with a positive outcome in the treatment of ITP.

Case 8

The history, together with the blood investigations, confirms a likely diagnosis of haemophilia, which is typically associated with a prolonged APTT. To differentiate between haemophilia A and B, one must undertake screening for deficiency of factor VIII and factor IX respectively. The treatment of haemophilia A relies on the use of factor VIII replacement and desmopressin. Haemophilia B management relies on factor IX replacement. The BCSH recommend that adolescents and adult patients with severe haemophilia A should take regular prophylaxis with factor VIII concentrates. Individuals on long-term treatment should have their regimens reviewed every 6 months. If no breakthrough bleeds have occurred, a trial of dose reduction is appropriate.

Case 9

The prolonged APTT and bleeding time point to a likely diagnosis of von Willebrand's disease (VWD). To confirm such a diagnosis, screening for von Willebrand factor is important.

The UK Haemophilia Centre Doctors' Organisation (UKHCDO) advises the use of desmopressin (DDAVP) in the first instance. For patients unresponsive to DDAVP, von Willebrand factor containing factor VIII concentrates are used, which include BPL 8Y, Haemate P, Alphanate and VHP VWF concentrate. Patients with VWD undergoing major surgery require coverage with desmopressin as a first-line treatment.

Case 10

The presence of a temperature and existence of neutropenia confirms a likely diagnosis of neutropenic sepsis. Management in accordance with NICE relies on the use of beta-lactam monotherapy with piperacillin and tazobactam. Further discussion on sepsis management is discussed in a previous case.

Case 11

The blood results indicate a likely diagnosis of disseminated intravascular coagulation (DIC). The International Society on Thrombosis and Haemostasis (ISTH) has devised a scoring system for DIC, which has demonstrated a close correlation with increasing mortality.

- Platelet count ($>100 \times 10^9$/L = 0, $<100 \times 10^9$/L =1, $<50 \times 10^9$/L = 2).
- Elevated fibrin marker (e.g. D-dimer, fibrin degradation products) (no increase = 0, moderate increase = 2, strong increase = 3).
- Prolonged PT (<3 s = 0, >3 but <6 s = 1, >6 s = 2).
- Fibrinogen level (>1 g/L = 0, <1 g/L = 1).

Score calculation

- ≥5 compatible with overt DIC: repeat score daily.
- <5 suggestive for non-overt DIC: repeat next 1–2 days.

The mainstay form of treatment relies on treatment of the underlying condition. The BCSH advises transfusion of platelets in patients with DIC and bleeding or at high risk of bleeding and a platelet count $<50 \times 10^9$/L. In non-bleeding patients with DIC, platelet transfusion is not advised. In bleeding patients with DIC and a prolonged PT and APTT, FFP may be useful. An alternative is prothrombin complex concentrate. Severely low levels of fibrinogen that persist despite FFP may be treated with fibrinogen concentrate or cryoprecipitate.

In cases of DIC where thrombosis is a major feature, heparin is advised. Patients with severe sepsis and DIC may benefit from recombinant human-activated protein C.

Case 12

The high white cell count and presence of blast cells within the bone marrow point to a diagnosis of acute myeloid leukaemia (AML). In acute lymphoblastic leukaemia (ALL), blast cells tend to be more prevalent in the peripheral blood. The treatment of AML relies heavily on chemotherapy, namely daunorubicin and cytarabine. The BCSH advises that rasburicase should be used in combination with chemotherapy for patients with hyperleucocytosis at risk of acute tumour lysis syndrome (a metabolic outcome of chemotherapy comprising hyperuricaemia, hyperphosphataemia, hyperkalaemia, hypocalcaemia and renal failure). Bone marrow transplantation is a salvage treatment in the event of relapse.

Case 13

The raised lymphocyte count and presence of smudge cells confirms a likely diagnosis of chronic lymphocytic leukaemia. Treatment depends on meeting the following National Cancer Institute criteria.

1   Progressive marrow failure: the development or worsening of anaemia and/or thrombocytopenia.
2   Massive (>10 cm) or progressive lymphadenopathy.
3   Massive (>6 cm) or progressive splenomegaly.
4   Progressive lymphocytosis >50% increase over 2 months.
5   Lymphocyte doubling time <6 months.
6   Systemic symptoms:*
    ‣ weight loss >10% in previous 6 months
    ‣ fever >38 °C for ≥2 weeks
    ‣ extreme fatigue
    ‣ night sweats
    ‣ autoimmune cytopenias.

*It is important to exclude other causes for these symptoms, such as infection.

According to the BCSH, initial treatment relies upon the use of chlorambucil. Those who then subsequently relapse may benefit from fludarabine. For those who become resistant to fludarabine, treatment options of choice include:
● High dose methylprednisolone and alemtuzumab.
● Younger individuals may benefit from an allogenic transplantation.
● Splenectomy can be utilised in cases of massive splenomegaly and refractory cytopenias.

Case 14

The history and examination together with the blood results point to a likely diagnosis of polycythaemia vera in view of the raised red cell mass, thrombocytosis, neutrophilia and splenomegaly. The management of polycythemia in accordance with the BCSH relies first and foremost on venesection aiming for a haematocrit of less than 0.45 L/L. Patients should be commenced on aspirin 75 mg daily in view of the thrombocytosis and cytoreduction should be considered in cases of:

- poor tolerance of venesection
- symptomatic or progressive splenomegaly
- other evidence of disease progression, e.g. weight loss and night sweats
- thrombocytosis.

The choice of cytoreduction is as follows:

- <40 years old: first-line interferon, second-line hydroxycarbamide or anagrelide;
- 40–75 years old: first-line hydroxycarbamide, second-line interferon or anagrelide;
- >75 years old: first-line hydroxycarbamide, second-line ^{32}P or intermittent low dose busulphan.

Case 15

The existence of teardrop-shaped red cells in addition to anaemia, a raised white cell and platelet count point to a diagnosis of myelofibrosis. In accordance with the BCSH, management focuses on the use of hydroxycarbamide, thalidomide and prednisolone. Splenectomy also has a well-established role in management and is indicated in cases of:

- drug refractory symptomatic splenomegaly
- drug refractory anaemia
- symptomatic portal hypertension
- catabolic symptoms including cachexia.

Radiotherapy is instigated in cases of severe bone pain, patients not suitable for surgical intervention and extramedullary haemopoiesis involving vital organs. Red cell transfusion is also recommended in cases of symptomatic anaemia. A trial of erythropoietin (EPO) can be used in anaemic patients with inappropriately low EPO levels. The androgen-based therapy danazol can be considered as an option to enhance the haemoglobin concentration of patients with myelofibrosis and transfusion-dependent anaemia. Research has shown that patients may benefit from allogenic stem cell transplantation as a curative option.

Case 16

In view of the history and investigations, the most likely diagnosis is multiple myeloma. The International Myeloma Working Group holds the following criteria to help distinguish between monoclonal gammopathy of undetermined significance (MGUS) and myeloma.

MGUS	Asymptomatic myeloma	Symptomatic myeloma
M-protein in serum <30 g/L	M-protein in serum >30 g/L and/or bone marrow clonal plasma cells >10%	M-protein in serum and/or urine
Bone marrow clonal plasma cells <10% and low level of plasma cell infiltration in a trephine biopsy (if done)		Bone marrow (clonal) plasma cells or biopsy-proven plasmacytoma
No related organ or tissue impairment (no end organ damage including bone lesions)	No related organ or tissue impairment (no end organ damage including bone lesions) or symptoms	Myeloma-related organ or tissue impairment (including bone lesions)

Myeloma related organ or tissue impairment refers to:

Increased calcium levels	Corrected serum calcium >0.25 mmol/L above the upper limit of normal or >2.75 mmol/L
Renal insufficiency	Creatinine >173 mmol/L
Anaemia	Haemoglobin 2 g/dL below the lower limit of normal or haemoglobin <10 g/dL
Bone lesions	Lytic lesions or osteoporosis with compression fractures (MRI or CT may clarify)
Other	Symptomatic hyperviscosity, amyloidosis, recurrent bacterial infections (>2 episodes in 12 months)

The main treatment of choice in multiple myeloma is chemotherapy and can comprise the following induction therapy:

- cyclophosphamide, thalidomide and dexamethasone (CTD)
- thalidomide, doxorubicin and dexamethasone (TAD), bortezomib/dexamethasone and bortezomib, doxorubicin and dexamethasone (PAD)
- autologous stem cell transplant is considered a useful treatment option in patients younger than 65 with adequate performance status and organ function.

Myeloma-related emergencies

Hyperviscosity is a common occurrence in myeloma and is best treated with therapeutic plasma exchange with saline fluid replacement. Hypercalcaemia is treated with fluids and bisphosphonates. Bisphosphonates are recommended in all cases of symptomatic multiple myeloma regardless of bone lesions. Bone pain benefits from the use of radiotherapy. In case of spinal cord compression, neurosurgical/oncological input is required and patients can benefit from decompression and radiotherapy.

8 Rheumatology

Case 1

The blood results demonstrate a positive ACPA, which is highly specific for rheumatoid arthritis (RA). The diagnosis of rheumatoid arthritis is based on the following American College of Rheumatology criteria.

A	1 large joint	0
	2–10 large joints	1
	1–3 small joints	2
	4–10 small joints	3
	>10 joints	5
B	Negative RF and negative ACPA	0
	Low-positive RF or low-positive ACPA	2
	High-positive RF or high-positive ACPA	3
C	Normal CRP and normal ESR	0
	Abnormal CRP or abnormal ESR	1
D	≤6 weeks symptom duration	0
	≥6 weeks symptom duration	1

Classification criteria for RA (score-based algorithm: add score of categories A–D; a score of ≥6/10 is needed for classification of a patient as having definite RA).

Once a diagnosis is made, NICE advocates the use of DMARDs and biologics such as anti-TNF-alpha inhibitors as soon as possible. The biologic anakinra is not routinely recommended in the treatment of RA. Commonly used DMARDs include hydroxychloroquine, leflunomide, methotrexate, mycophenolate mofetil (MMF), D-penicillamine and sulphasalazine. Glucocorticoids are utilised for the treatment of rheumatoid flares. Symptom control should be sought through NSAIDs or COX-2 inhibitors.

The requirement for surgical intervention relies upon:
- persistent pain because of joint damage or other soft-tissue cause
- worsening joint function
- progressive deformity
- persistent localised synovitis
- imminent or actual tendon rupture
- nerve compression
- stress fracture

- suspected or proven septic arthritis
- symptoms or signs suggesting cervical myelopathy.

It is also advised that patients with RA should be offered multidisciplinary input in the form of occupational therapy and physiotherapy.

Case 2

The joint aspirate is in keeping with septic arthritis. Additional investigations include polarising microscopy. In addition, blood cultures should be taken, and bloods should be sent for white cell count, ESR and CRP. The British Society for Rheumatology Standards working group advise that imaging has no role in the diagnosis of septic arthritis. Antibiotics of choice are as follows:

No risk factors for atypical organisms	Flucloxacillin 2 g qds IV. Local policy may be to add gentamicin IV. If penicillin allergic, clindamycin 450–600 mg qds IV or 2nd or 3rd generation cephalosporin IV
High risk of Gram-negative sepsis (elderly, frail, recurrent UTI, and recent abdominal surgery)	2nd or 3rd generation cephalosporin, e.g. cefuroxime 1.5 g tds IV. Local policy may be to add flucloxacillin IV to 3rd generation cephalosporin Discuss allergic patients with microbiology – Gram stain may influence antibiotic choice
MRSA risk (known MRSA, recent inpatient, nursing home resident, leg ulcers or catheters, or other risk factors determined locally)	Vancomycin IV plus 2nd or 3rd generation cephalosporin IV
Suspected gonococcus or meningococcus	Ceftriaxone IV or similar, dependent on local policy or resistance

It is important to note that septic joints should be aspirated to dryness as often as is required.

Case 3

In view of the negatively birefringent urate crystals the diagnosis here is gout. Serum urate may be normal in 10% of cases of gout. In the acute phase, the British Society for Rheumatology (BSR) advises the use of NSAIDs. Colchicine is an effective alternative but is slower to work. Intra-articular corticosteroids are also highly effective in acute attacks. Allopurinol should not be commenced during an acute attack. Patients should also be watchful of their weight, restrict purine-containing foods as well as alcohol.

Case 4

In view of the history and investigations, the most likely diagnosis is systemic lupus erythematosus (SLE). The diagnosis is based on satisfying four of the clinical and immunological criteria in the Systemic Lupus International Collaborating Clinics (SLICC) classification criteria, including at least one clinical criterion and one immunological criterion, OR if she has biopsy-proven nephritis compatible with SLE in the presence of ANAs or anti-dsDNA antibodies.

Clinical criteria

Acute cutaneous lupus

Chronic cutaneous lupus

Oral ulcers

Non-scarring alopecia

Synovitis

Serositis

Renal – urine protein–creatinine ratio (or 24-hour urine protein) representing 500 mg protein/24 hours
OR red blood cell casts

Neurological involvement

Haemolytic anaemia

Leukopenia

Thrombocytopenia

Immunological criteria

ANA

Anti-double stranded DNA

Anti-smooth muscle antibody

Antiphospholipid antibody

Low complement

Direct Coomb's test

The management relies upon the use of anti-malarials and glucocorticoids. Those patients who are non-responsive benefit from the use of azathioprine, MMF and methotrexate. Photo protection should be considered for those with skin manifestations.

Case 5

In view of the history and positive anti-centromere and Scl-70 antibodies, the most likely diagnosis is systemic sclerosis. The European League Against Rheumatism (EULAR) advises the use of nifedipine and iloprost in cases of Raynaud's phenomenon associated attacks. Individuals with digital ulcers should be treated with iloprost. Bosentan may be useful in the treatment of ulcers in diffuse systemic sclerosis. Those with associated pulmonary artery hypertension may benefit from bosentan, sitaxentan, sildenafil, as well as epoprostenol. For skin involvement, methotrexate is a worthwhile agent. Cyclophosphamide should be used in the treatment of interstitial lung disease. For renal crises, ACE inhibitors may prove beneficial. For GI-related disease, patients may benefit from PPIs, prokinetics and antibiotics in cases of bacterial overgrowth.

Case 6

In view of the patient's presentation and positive anti Mi-2 antibodies the most likely diagnosis is dermatomyositis. The treatment of choice is steroids in addition to other immunosuppressives such as methotrexate and azathioprine. Research also demonstrates some benefit through the use of IvIg. Skin complaints may benefit from the use of hydroxychloroquine.

Case 7

Taking into account the presentation and positive PR3 ANCA findings, the most likely diagnosis is Wegener's granulomatosis (WG). The BSR advises the following treatment regimen for WG which applies to all primary vasculitides in general. For localised disease/creatinine <150 mcmol/L, prednisolone and methotrexate or cyclophosphamide should be commenced. For generalised/organ-threatening disease with a serum creatinine <500 mcmol/L, prednisolone and cyclophosphamide should be started. For severe/life-threatening disease with a serum creatinine >500 mcmol/L, prednisolone and cyclophosphamide in addition to plasma exchange should be commenced. Once in remission, prednisolone can be tapered with a switch to azathioprine or methotrexate, which are then also slowly reduced accordingly.

9 Respiratory

Case 1

The chest X-ray demonstrates evidence of right lower zone atelectasis with left lower lobe consolidation as well as a left-sided pleural effusion. Compare this X-ray with the one below demonstrating evidence of bilateral pleural effusions.

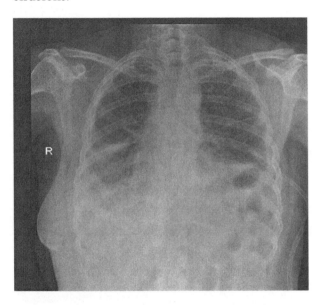

Here is another chest X-ray demonstrating evidence of pneumonia:

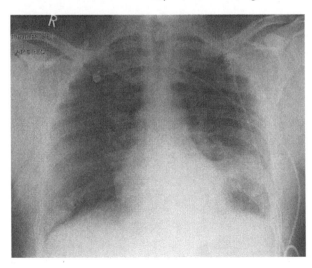

Here you can see large cavitating lesions in the right-lower, left-mid and left-lower zones. Cavitating lesions are most likely seen in cases of pneumonia due to *Klebsiella* and *Staphylococcus aureus*.

In cases of pneumonia, it is important to request the following blood investigations: white cell count and CRP, urea and electrolytes and liver function tests. Inflammatory markers as a general rule are important in all cases of infection. Individuals with pneumonia are often dehydrated and hence assessment of renal function is key. In addition, legionella pneumonia can often cause hyponatremia. Deranged liver function can be seen in atypical pneumonia cases such as mycoplasma. An arterial blood gas is key as it helps to determine the degree of hypoxia and acidosis. Severely hypoxic patients may require intubation and patients with type II respiratory failure often require non-invasive ventilation (NIV). Blood cultures are an additional investigation of importance and should ideally be obtained before starting antibiotics. Sputum should be sent for microscopy and culture. Urine should also be sent for *Legionella* and *Streptococcus pneumoniae*.

The pleural effusion is in this case most likely due to the pneumonia. A pleural aspiration under ultrasound guidance is essential to help exclude an empyema. A pleural effusion is classified as an exudate if any of the following Light's criteria are met:

- ratio of pleural fluid protein to serum protein greater than 0.5
- ratio of pleural fluid LDH to serum LDH greater than 0.6
- pleural fluid LDH greater than two-thirds of the upper limit of normal serum value.

Pleural fluid should ideally be sent for measurement of LDH, protein, glucose, pH, cell count, culture and cytology. If the pH of the pleural fluid is less than 7.2 the effusion is an empyema and requires drainage. A CT scan is essential in all cases of a pleural effusion. If malignancy is suspected, then a pleural biopsy is needed. A thoracoscopy is advised in cases where the effusion is an exudate and malignancy is suspected.

From the case described, the patient is hypotensive and tachycardic secondary to sepsis. Urgent fluid resuscitation is required typically with colloids. In view of his low oxygen saturations, high flow oxygen is important. Oxygen therapy should be tailored in order to achieve a PO_2 of more than 8 kPa and oxygen saturations of between 94%–98%. Patients who are severely septic are often immobile in hospital and will require venous thromboprophylaxis.

The use of antibiotics is the mainstay form of treatment for pneumonia.

Antibiotics are given according to severity, which is based on the CURB-65 criteria:

C – confusion
U – urea > 7 mmol/L
R – respiratory rate > 30 breaths per minute
B – blood pressure less than 90 mmHg systolic
Age > 65

According to the British Thoracic Society (BTS), the following treatment regime is advised:

Severity	CURB-65 score	Treatment
Low severity	0–1	Amoxicillin orally
Moderate severity	2	Amoxicillin plus clarithromycin orally or IV
High severity	3–5	Co-amoxiclav plus clarithromycin IV

Patients with low or moderately severe pneumonia require 7 days of anti-biotics typically and patients with high severity pneumonia may require up to 10–14 days of treatment.

With regard to a malignant pleural effusion, management as per BTS guidelines relies upon aspiration, chest drain insertion and pleurodesis with consideration of an indwelling pleural catheter.

Case 2

The chest X-ray demonstrates evidence of miliary opacifications bilaterally consistent with miliary TB.

Of course miliary TB is fairly easy to spot – TB on a chest X-ray may present in a variety of ways such as cavity formation, infiltrates or calcified nodules (see below X-ray).

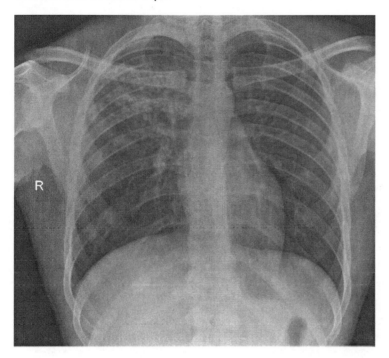

In cases of suspected TB, sputum should be sent for culture on three consecutive days. Blood investigations are also important, in particular white cell count, CRP, liver function tests and HIV serology.

A Mantoux test is the primary test for latent TB. It involves injection of tuberculin purified protein derivative (PPD) and measurement of the subsequent induration. An induration of 5 mm or less is deemed a negative result. Interferon gamma testing should take place for people with positive Mantoux testing and in people whose Mantoux testing may be less reliable.

According to NICE, the management of respiratory TB requires a 6-month regimen of isoniazid, rifampicin (6 months), pyrazinamide and ethambutol (for the first 2 months only). Patients should remain in hospital for treatment for at least 2 weeks before being discharged for outpatient management.

Case 3

The chest X-ray demonstrates evidence of pulmonary fibrosis.

In addition to a chest X-ray, a high resolution CT is both sensitive and specific for pulmonary fibrosis (see CT below). Lung function tests are often useful and demonstrate a restrictive lung defect. If the diagnosis remains unclear after imaging, a transbronchial lung biopsy is the next investigative procedure of choice.

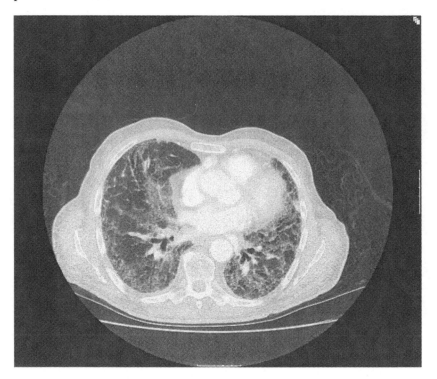

High resolution CT demonstrating evidence of honeycombing and reticular opacities.

There is no gold standard treatment for pulmonary fibrosis. Patients benefit from oxygen therapy, pulmonary rehabilitation and opiates. The British Thoracic Society advises the use of prednisolone, azathioprine and N-acetylcysteine. Patients should be referred to a lung transplant centre if their disease is advanced, i.e TLCO is <40% predicted or is progressive, i.e >10% decline in FVC.

Case 4

The chest X-ray demonstrates evidence of hyperinflation and bullae in the left upper zone in keeping with chronic obstructive pulmonary disease (COPD).

An arterial blood gas is essential in all patients presenting with an exacerbation of COPD. Patients with evidence of type II respiratory failure require NIV. Blood investigations rely on measurement of the white cell count, CRP, as well as urea and electrolytes. Serum potassium monitoring is particularly important due to the risk of hypokalaemia secondary to beta agonists and theophylline. Sputum should also be sent for microscopy and culture as well as blood cultures if the patient is pyrexial. Lung function tests help to determine the severity of airflow obstruction, which is non-reversible. According to NICE, the following severity criteria is utilised:

Stage 1	Mild FEV1	>80% predicted
Stage 2	Moderate FEV1	50%–79% predicted
Stage 3	Severe FEV1	30%–49% predicted
Stage 4	Very severe	<30% predicted

In addition to a chest X-ray, a chest CT is particularly useful for diagnosing emphysema.

The management of an exacerbation of COPD relies on the use of careful oxygen therapy, aiming typically for saturations of 88%–92%. Bronchodilators and steroids are the mainstay form of treatment. Antibiotics used are of the penicillin or tetracycline class. Prednisolone at a dose of 30 mg daily is the most appropriate steroid of choice for a maximum of 7–14 days. According to NICE, intravenous theophylline is useful in cases where response to nebulised bronchodilators is inadequate.

NIV is often employed in cases where there is persistent hypercapnic failure despite optimum medical therapy.

Case 5

The chest X-ray demonstrates a large left-sided pneumothorax.

In addition to a chest X-ray, a CT chest may be particularly useful. Such an investigation is of course not routinely done in the acute setting but can be used to help aid diagnosis, for example in distinguishing between bullous disease and a pneumothorax.

Patients presenting with a pneumothorax should be given adequate oxygenation and analgesia as needed.

The British Thoracic Society advises the following with regard to the management of a pneumothorax:

1   If <2 cm and/or breathless, for aspiration.
2   If >2 cm and/or breathless, for chest drain insertion.

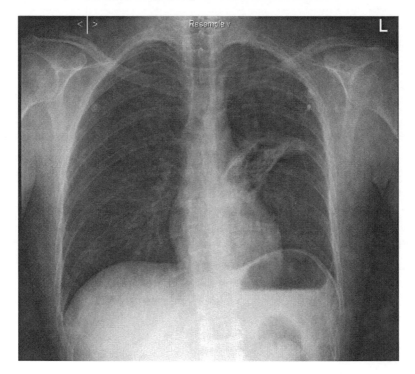

And, in case you were wondering, here is the chest X-ray following insertion of a chest drain. There are new atelectatic changes in the left-mid zone compared to the initial chest X-ray.

Case 6

The chest X-ray demonstrates evidence of bilateral reticulonodular infiltration in keeping with extrinsic allergic alveolitis (hypersensitivity pneumonitis).

Blood investigations, in particular ESR and serum preciptins are particularly useful tests. A high resolution CT will show ground glass opacities. Lung function tests are also worthwhile and will demonstrate a restrictive lung defect.

The most likely precipitant in this case is mouldy hay in view of the patient's occupation. Avoidance of the precipitant in question is key to management. The use of steroids has been shown to be useful in treating severe or progressive disease.

Case 7

The chest X-ray shows evidence of prominence of the left hilum.

Taking into account the history, examination and chest X-ray findings, one must exclude the possibility of lung cancer. Useful investigations therefore include a serum calcium and liver function tests. Serum calcium may be raised secondary to excess production of parathyroid hormone, parathyroid hormone related peptide or simply due to bone metastases. Liver function tests may be deranged secondary to liver metastases. Sputum should be sent for cytology and a chest CT should be performed for staging purposes. A bronchoscopy is key as it allows for a tissue diagnosis. It is important to note that cancer can only be confirmed following histological confirmation and one can only ever be suspicious of cancer from imaging. If in the case of an unconfirmed diagnosis following bronchoscopy or CT-guided biopsy, a thoracoscopy is the next useful investigation. PET scanning is reserved for cases of solitary pulmonary nodules or assessing extent of spread.

According to NICE, patients with non-small cell lung cancer are treated surgically in the first instance. Radiotherapy is indicated for stage I, II and III disease. Chemotherapy is offered for patients with more severe disease, namely stage III or IV disease.

With regard to small cell lung cancer, the treatment of choice is chemotherapy.

A detailed overview of lung cancer staging is beyond the scope of this book but can be obtained from the American Joint Committee on Cancer, available at www.cancerstaging.org.

Case 8

The arterial blood gas demonstrates evidence of significant hypoxia with a non-compensated respiratory alkalosis. Together with the history and examination findings the most likely diagnosis is asthma. In the acute phase as patients are hyperventilating they 'blow off' their CO_2. As the patient tires their respiratory effort decreases and they are at risk of type II respiratory failure.

To exclude an underlying chest infection or pneumothorax, a chest X-ray is essential. Peak flow assessment is also of particular importance. To confirm a suspected diagnosis of asthma in the non-acute setting, spirometry is key, demonstrating an obstructive defect with reversibility being noted by an increase in FEV1 by 15% following bronchodilator therapy.

The management of asthma in an acute setting is severity dependent. According to the British Thoracic Society, asthma is graded as follows:

Severity	Features
Moderate	Worsening symptoms PEF > 50%–75% predicted No features of acute severe asthma
Acute severe	PEF 33%–50% predicted Respiratory rate > 25 breaths per minute Heart rate > 110 beats per minute Inability to complete sentences in one breath
Life-threatening	PEF < 33% predicted Oxygen saturations < 92% PO_2 < 8 kPa Normal PCO_2 Silent chest Cyanosis Poor respiratory effort Arrhythmias Exhaustion
Near fatal	Raised PCO_2 and/or requiring mechanical ventilation

Management relies on adequate oxygenation with a saturation aim of between 94%–98%. Nebulised bronchodilators (salbutamol and ipratropium bromide) and steroids (prednisolone 40–50 mg daily) are essential. In acute severe, life-threatening, or fatal asthma IV magnesium sulphate should be given.

Patients with deteriorating peak flow, persistent hypoxia and hypercapnea require intensive care input.

Case 9

The ECG demonstrates right bundle branch block. Together with the history the most likely diagnosis is a pulmonary embolus.

Patients with a suspected PE should undergo an arterial blood gas to assess the degree of hypoxia. D-dimer measurement is also important and if negative helps to reliably exclude a PE. According to the BTS, a CTPA is the recommended imaging modality for non-massive and massive PEs. An ECHO will also help to confirm the diagnosis of a massive PE. Isotope lung scanning is undertaken in patients without underlying cardiac or pulmonary disease and in those where the initial chest X-ray is deemed normal. Based on these criteria, if the isotope lung scan is normal, a PE can be excluded.

According to the BTS, thrombolysis with 50 mg alteplase is the first-line treatment for a massive PE. In all other cases, low molecular weight heparin should be considered initially if a PE is suspected. Once a PE has been confirmed, oral anticoagulation with warfarin is commenced aiming for an INR of between 2 and 3. Such treatment is continued for up to 6 weeks for temporary risk factors, 3 months for idiopathic first cases and for 6 months in all other cases. IVC filters are employed in cases where anticoagulation is contraindicated or unsuccessful in preventing a recurrence of PE from DVTs.

References

1 Cardiology

- Maisch B, Seferović PM, Ristić AD *et al.* Guidelines on the diagnosis and management of pericardial diseases. ESC guidelines. *Eur Heart J.* 2004; **25**: 587–610. Available at: www.escardio.org/guidelines-surveys/esc-guidelines/Pages/pericardial-diseases.aspx.
- National Institute for Health and Clinical Excellence. *Chronic Heart Failure: NICE guideline 108.* London: NIHCE; 2010. www.nice.org.uk/CG108.
- National Institute for Health and Clinical Excellence. *Hypertension: NICE guideline 127.* London: NIHCE; 2011. http://guidance.nice.org.uk/CG127.
- National Institute for Health and Clinical Excellence. *The Management of Atrial Fibrillation: NICE guideline 36.* London: NIHCE; 2006. www.nice.org.uk/CG36.
- Resuscitation Council (UK). Resuscitation guidelines. Available at: www.resus.org.uk.
- Scottish Intercollegiate Guidelines Network. *Acute Coronary Syndrome: SIGN guideline 93.* Edinburgh: SIGN; 2013. www.sign.ac.uk/guidelines/fulltext/93/index.html.

2 Endocrinology

- Joint British Diabetes Societies Inpatient Care Group. *The Management of Diabetic Ketoacidosis in Adults.* JBDS IP Group; Mar 2010. Available at: www.diabetes.org.uk.
- Joint British Diabetes Societies Inpatient Care Group. *The Management of the Hyperosmolar Hyperglycaemic State (HHS) in Adults with Diabetes.* JBDS IP Group; Aug 2012. Available at: www.diabetes.nhs.uk.
- National Institute for Health and Clinical Excellence. *Type 2 Diabetes: NICE guideline 66.* London: NIHCE; 2008. http://guidance.nice.org.uk/CG66.
- The Endocrine Society. *The Diagnosis of Cushing's Syndrome.* The Endocrine Society; 2008. Available at: www.endo-society.org/guidelines/final/upload/Cushings_Guideline.pdf.
- World Health Organization. *Definition and Diagnosis of Diabetes Mellitus and Intermediate Hyperglycaemia.* Geneva: WHO; 2006. Available at: www.who.int/diabetes/publications/diagnosis_diabetes2006/en/index.html.

3 Gastroenterology

- Bauer MP, Kuijper EJ, van Dissel JT. Treatment guidance document for *Clostridium difficile* infection. *Clin Microbiol Infect.* 2009; **15**: 1067–79.

Available at: www.escmid.org/escmid_library/medical_guidelines/
escmid_guidelines/#c3762.

- Gleeson D, Heneghan MA. Guidelines for the management of autoimmune hepatitis. BSG guideline. *Gut*. 2011; **60**: 1611–29. Available at: www.bsg.org.uk/clinical-guidelines/Liver/guidelines-for-the-management-of-autoimmune-hepatitis.html.

- Hepatitis B management. CKS NHS. Available at: www.cks.nhs.uk/hepatitis_b/management/scenario_diagnosis/interpretation_of_serology_tests/interpretation_of_hepatitis_b_serology_tests_table.

- Mowat C, Cole A, Windsor A *et al.* Guidelines for the management of inflammatory bowel disease in adults. BSG guideline. *Gut*. 2011. Available at: www.bsg.org.uk/clinical-guidelines/ibd/guidelines-for-the-management-of-inflammatory-bowel-disease.html.

- National Institute for Health and Clinical Excellence. *Acute Upper GI Bleeding: NICE guideline 141*. London: NIHCE; 2012. http://guidance.nice.org.uk/CG141.

- National Institute for Health and Clinical Excellence. *Dyspepsia: NICE guideline 17*. London: NIHCE; 2004. http://guidance.nice.org.uk/CG17.

- Ryder SD. Guidelines for the diagnosis and treatment of hepatocellular carcinoma (HCC) in adults. BSG guideline. *Gut*. 2003; **52**(Suppl. 3): S1–8. Available at: www.bsg.org.uk/clinical-guidelines/Liver/guidelines-for-the-diagnosis-and-treatment-of-hepatocellular-carcinoma-hcc-in-adults.html.

- Lee WM, Larson AM, Stravitz RT. The management of acute liver failure. *Hepatology*. September 2011; 1–22. Available at: www.aasld.org/practiceguidelines/Documents/AcuteLiverFailureUpdate2011.pdf.

- Truelove SC, Witts LJ. Cortisone in ulcerative colitis: final report on a therapeutic trial. *Br Med J*. 1955; **2**: 1041–8.

- UK Working Party on Acute Pancreatitis. UK guidelines for the management of acute pancreatitis. BSG guideline. *Gut*. 2005; **54**(Suppl. 3): S1–9. Available at: www.bsg.org.uk/pdf_word_docs/pancreatic.pdf.

4 Neurology

- Association of British Neurologists. *ABN Revised (2009) Guidelines for Prescribing in Multiple Sclerosis*. London: ABN; 2009. Available at: www.theabn.org/Newsdetails.aspx?news=428.

- Dellinger RP, Levy MM, Rhodes A *et al.* Surviving Sepsis Campaign: international guidelines for management of severe sepsis and septic shock. *Crit Care Med*. 2013; **41**(2): 580–637. Available at: www.survivingsepsis.org/guidelines/Pages/default.aspx.

- National Institute for Health and Clinical Excellence. *Multiple Sclerosis: NICE guideline 8*. London: NIHCE; 2003. Available at http://guidance.nice.org.uk/CG8.

- National Institute for Health and Clinical Excellence. *Stroke: NICE guideline 68*. London: NIHCE; 2008. Available at www.nice.org.uk/cg68.

5 Overdose

- Dargan P, Wallace CI, Jones AL. An evidence based flowchart to guide the management of acute salicylate (aspirin) overdose. *Emerg Med J.* 2002; **19**: 206–9.
- MHRA. *Paracetamol overdose.* Available at: www.mhra.gov.uk.
- O'Grady J, Alexander G, Hayllar K *et al.* Early indicators of prognosis in fulminant hepatic failure. *Gastroenterology.* 1989; **97**(2): 439–45.

6 Renal

- Lewington A, Kanagasundaram S. *Acute kidney injury.* The Renal Association; 2011. Available at: www.renal.org/clinical/guidelinessection/AcuteKidneyInjury. aspx.
- National Institute for Health and Clinical Excellence. *Chronic Kidney Disease: NICE guideline 73.* London: NIHCE; 2008. www.nice.org.uk/CG073.
- National Institute for Health and Clinical Excellence. *Familial Hypercholesterolaemia: quick reference guide. NICE guideline 71.* London: NIHCE; 2008. http://guidance.nice.org.uk/CG71/QuickRefGuide/pdf/English.

7 Haematology

- British Committee for Standards in Haematology and UK Myeloma Forum. Guidelines on the diagnosis and management of multiple myeloma. BCSH guidelines. 2010. Available at: www.bcshguidelines.com/documents/ MYELOMA_Mngmt_GUIDELINE_REVISION_Sept_2010.pdf.
- Guidelines for the diagnosis and management of disseminated intravascular coagulation. BCSH guidelines. *Br J Haematol.* 2009; **145**: 24–33. Available at: www.bcshguidelines.com.
- McMullin MF, Bareford D, Campbell P *et al.* Guidelines for the diagnosis, investigation and management of polycythaemia/erythrocytosis. BCSH guidelines. *Br J Haematol.* 2005; **130**: 174–95. Available at: www.bcshguidelines. com/documents/polycythaemia_bjh_2005.pdf.
- Milligan DW, Grimwade D, Cullis JO *et al.* Guidelines on the management of acute myeloid leukaemia. BCSH guidelines. *Br J Haematol.* 2006; **135**: 450–74. Available at: www.bcshguidelines.com/documents/aml_bjh_2006.pdf.
- National Institute for Health and Clinical Excellence. *Neutropenic Sepsis: NICE guideline 151.* London: NIHCE; 2012. http://guidance.nice.org.uk/CG151.
- Oscier D, Fegan C, Hillmen P *et al.* Guidelines on the diagnosis and management of chronic lymphocytic leukaemia. BCSH guidelines. *Br J Haematol.* 2004; **125**: 294–317. Available at: www.bcshguidelines.com/documents/ chronicLL_05052004.pdf.
- Pasi KJ, Collins PW, Keeling DM *et al.* Management of von Willebrand disease: a guideline from the UK Haemophilia Centre Doctors' Organization. *Haemophilia.* 2004; **10**(3): 218–31. Available at: www.ukhcdo.org/UKHCDOguidelines.htm.
- Rees DC, Olujohungbe AD, Parker NE *et al.* Guidelines for the management of the acute painful crisis in sickle cell disease. BCSH guidelines. *Br J Haematol.*

2003; **120**: 744–52. Available at: www.bcshguidelines.com/documents/ sicklecelldisease_bjh_2003.pdf.

- Reilly JT, McMullin MF, Beer PA *et al*. Guidelines for the diagnosis and management of myelofibrosis. BCSH guideline. Available at: www.bcshguidelines. com/documents/PMF_Guidelines_16_(CLEAN).pdf.
- Richards M, Williams M, Chalmers E *et al*. Guideline on the use of prophylactic factor VIII concentrate in children and adults with severe haemophilia A. BCSH guidelines. *Br J Haematol*. 2010; **149**: 498–507. Available at: www.bcshguidelines. com/documents/prophylactic_facto_viiirbjh_04_2010.pdf.

8 Rheumatology

- Aletaha D, Neogi T, Silman AJ *et al*. 2010 Rheumatoid arthritis classification criteria. *Arthritis Rheum*. 2010; **62**(9): 2569–81. Available at: www.rheumatology. org/practice/clinical/classification/ra/2010_revised_criteria_classification_ra.pdf.
- Coakley G, Mathews C, Field M *et al*. BSR & BHPR, BOA, RCGP and BSAC guidelines for management of the hot swollen joint in adults. *Rheumatology*. 2006; **45**(8): 1039–41. Available at: http://rheumatology.oxfordjournals.org/ content/45/8/1039.full.pdf+html.
- Jordan KM, Cameron JS, Snaith M *et al*. British Society for Rheumatology and British Health Professionals in Rheumatology Guideline for the Management of Gout. *Rheumatology*. 2007; **46**(8): 1372–4. Available at: www.rheumatology.org. uk/includes/documents/cm_docs/2009/m/management_of_gout.pdf.
- Kowal-Bielecka O, Landewé R, Avouac J *et al*. EULAR recommendations for the treatment of systemic sclerosis: a report from the EULAR Scleroderma Trials and Research group (EUSTAR). *Ann Rheum Dis*. 2009; **68**(5): 620–8.
- Lapraik C, Watts R, Bacon P *et al*. Management of adults with ANCA associated vasculitis. BSR guidelines. *Rheumatology*. 2007; **46**: 1–11. Available at: www. rheumatology.org.uk/resources/guidelines/bsr_guidelines.aspx.
- National Institute for Health and Clinical Excellence. *Rheumatoid Arthritis: NICE guideline 79*. London: NIHCE; 2009. www.nice.org.uk/CG79.
- Petri M, Orbai AM, Alarcón GS *et al*. Derivation and validation of the Systemic Lupus International Collaborating Clinics classification criteria for systemic lupus erythematosus. *Arthritis Rheum*. 2012; **64**: 2677–86.

9 Respiratory

- British Thoracic Society. *Asthma Guidelines*. Available at: www.brit-thoracic.org. uk/guidelines/asthma-guidelines.aspx.
- British Thoracic Society. Pleural disease guidelines 2010. *Thorax*. 2010; **65**(Suppl. 2). Available at: www.brit-thoracic.org.uk/guidelines/pleural-disease-guidelines-2010.aspx.
- British Thoracic Society. *Pulmonary Embolism Guidelines*. Available at: www.brit-thoracic.org.uk/guidelines/pulmonary-embolism-guidelines.aspx.
- Light R, Macgregor M, Luchsinger P *et al*. Pleural effusions: the diagnostic separation of transudates and exudates. *Ann Intern Med*. 1972; **77**(4): 507–13.

- Lim WS, Baudouin SV, George RC *et al*. Guidelines for the management of community acquired pneumonia in adults: update 2009. *Thorax*. 2009; **64**(Suppl. 3): S1–55. Available at: www.brit-thoracic.org.uk/guidelines/pneumonia-guidelines.aspx.
- National Institute for Health and Clinical Excellence. *Chronic Obstructive Pulmonary Disease: NICE guideline 101*. London: NIHCE; 2010. http://guidance.nice.org.uk/CG101.
- National Institute for Health and Clinical Excellence. *Lung Cancer: NICE guideline 121*. London: NIHCE; 2011. http://guidance.nice.org.uk/cg121.
- National Institute for Health and Clinical Excellence. *Tuberculosis: NICE guideline 117*. London: NIHCE; 2011. http://guidance.nice.org.uk/CG117.
- Wells AU, Hirani N. Interstitial lung disease guideline: the British Thoracic Society in collaboration with the Thoracic Society of Australia and New Zealand and the Irish Thoracic Society. *Thorax*. 2008; **63**(Suppl. 5): S1–58. Available at: www.brit-thoracic.org.uk/guidelines/interstitial-lung-disease-(dpld)-guideline.aspx.

Index

Figures and tables are indicated by locators in **bold**.

CPD with Radcliffe

You can now use a selection of our books to achieve CPD (Continuing Professional Development) points through directed reading.

We provide a free online form and downloadable certificate for your appraisal portfolio. Look for the CPD logo and register with us at: www.radcliffehealth.com/cpd

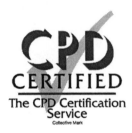